T0177521

OXFORD MEDICAL PUBLICATIONS

Oxford Specialist Handbooks
in Pain Medicine

Spinal Interventions in Pain Management

Oxford Specialist
Handbooks in
Pain Medicine

Spinal
Interventions
in Pain
Management

Edited by

Karen Simpson
Consultant in Pain Medicine
Leeds Teaching Hospitals NHS Trust, Leeds, UK

Ganesan Baranidharan
Consultant in Anaesthesia and Pain Medicine
Leeds Teaching Hospitals NHS Trust, Leeds, UK

Sanjeeva Gupta
Consultant in Pain Medicine and Anaesthesia
Bradford Teaching Hospitals NHS Foundation Trust
Bradford Royal Infirmary, Bradford, UK

Illustrations by

Simon Tordoff
Consultant in Anaesthesia and Pain Management
University Hospitals of Leicester NHS Trust
Leicester General Hospital, Leicester, UK

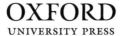

OXFORD
UNIVERSITY PRESS

OXFORD
UNIVERSITY PRESS

Great Clarendon Street, Oxford OX2 6DP

Oxford University Press is a department of the University of Oxford.
It furthers the University's objective of excellence in research, scholarship,
and education by publishing worldwide in

Oxford New York

Auckland Cape Town Dar es Salaam Hong Kong Karachi
Kuala Lumpur Madrid Melbourne Mexico City Nairobi
New Delhi Shanghai Taipei Toronto

With offices in

Argentina Austria Brazil Chile Czech Republic France Greece
Guatemala Hungary Italy Japan Poland Portugal Singapore
South Korea Switzerland Thailand Turkey Ukraine Vietnam

Oxford is a registered trade mark of Oxford University Press
in the UK and in certain other countries

Published in the United States
by Oxford University Press Inc., New York

British Library Cataloguing in Publication Data
Data available

Library of Congress Cataloging in Publication Data
Data available

Typeset by Cenveo, Bangalore, India
Printed in China on acid-free paper by
C&C Offset Printing Co., Ltd

ISBN 978–0–19–958691–2

10 9 8 7 6 5 4 3 2

Preface

The practice of pain medicine requires acquisition of the appropriate knowledge, skills, and attitudes to enable assessment and management of patients with a variety of acute, chronic, and cancer pains. Most countries have defined the curriculum for pain medicine within their national standard setting frameworks. The authors of this book assume that readers will already have had such an education. This book is focused on techniques rather than pain pathology, assessment, or treatment planning. This is not a book about theory or evidence for different interventions. These data emerge and evolve, and this information can be found in current journals. This is a practical handbook about applied anatomy, imaging, how to choose patients, and how to perform procedures accurately and safely; it includes pitfalls and pearls of wisdom from experts with many years of combined experience. The contributors all regularly perform the procedures that they describe. We hope that established pain specialists and trainees will dip into the chapters before planning a procedure and/or before an examination!

This book is multi-author—there are contributions from those with a national reputation for expertise in their area. The text covers most interventions for pain and includes neuromodulation (spinal cord stimulation and intrathecal drug delivery). The authors make reference to guidance from a variety of sources, e.g. the Faculty of Pain Medicine of the Royal College of Anaesthetists (UK), the Association of Anaesthetists (UK), the British Pain Society, the International Spine Intervention Society (USA), the International Neuromodulation Society (USA), and the American Society of Interventional Pain Physicians (USA). These bodies provide many useful clinical guidelines and web-based information for practitioners and patients, and we commend them to you.

The text is well illustrated with radiographs and figures; we are grateful to our authors for collecting, editing, and providing these. We are also indebted to patients for their permission to include them in the book. In addition, we are privileged to have drawings from Simon Tordoff whose artwork is a legend in the UK pain world. We would also like to thank our secretary Paula Harrison whose help in editing the final text was so welcome. Finally, we are grateful to our contributors for their diligence in writing for us and their commitment to excellence and detail.

Ganesan Baranidiharan
Sanjeeva Gupta
Karen H. Simpson
2011

Contents

Detailed contents

Contributors

Andrew Baker, MB ChB, FRCA

Specialty Registrar, St James's University Hospital, Beckett Street, Leeds, UK

Dr Shyam Balasubramanian

Consultant in Pain Management and Anaesthesia, Clinical Lead in Pain Medicine, University Hospitals Coventry and Warwickshire NHS Trust, Coventry, UK

Dr Ganesan Baranidharan

Consultant in Anaesthesia and Pain Medicine, Leeds Teaching Hospitals NHS Trust Leeds, UK

Dr Dudley Bush

Consultant Anaesthetist with an interest in pain management, Leeds Teaching Hospitals NHS Trust, Leeds, UK

Dr Muthusamy Chandramohan, MBBS, DMRD, FRCR

Consultant Musculoskeletal Radiologist, Bradford, UK

Dr Neil T Collighan

Consultant in Anaesthesia and Pain Management, East Kent Hospitals University Foundation NHS Trust, QEQM Hospital, St. Peter's Road, Margate, UK

Dr AR Cooper

Consultant in Anaesthesia and Pain Relief, Pain Relief Clinic, Causeway Hospital, 4 Newbridge Road, Coleraine, Co. Londonderry, UK

Sangeeta Das MBBS, DA, FRCA

Specialty Registrar, Anaesthetics, Bradford Royal Infirmary, Duckworth Lane, Bradford, UK

Dr Karthikeyan Dhandapani MBBS, DA, FCARCSI, FRCA

Specialty Registrar, Department of Anaesthesia, Leeds Teaching Hospital NHS Trust, Beckett Street, Leeds, UK

Dr Sam Eldabe, FRCA, FFPMRCA

Honorary Senior Lecturer, Cardiff University, and Consultant in Anaesthesia and Pain Management, Department of Pain and Anaesthesia, The James Cook University Hospital, Marton Road, Middlesbrough, UK

Dr Neal Evans

Consultant Pain Specialist, Wycombe General Hospital, Queen Alexandra Road, High Wycombe, Bucks, UK The Back Pain Team Ltd, The Paddocks Clinic, Aylesbury Road, Princes Risborough, Bucks, UK

Dr Clare Groves

Consultant Musculoskeletal Radiologist, Bradford, UK

Dr Ashish Gulve

Consultant in Pain Management and Anaesthesia, The James Cook University Hospital, Middlesbrough, UK

Dr Sanjeeva Gupta
Consultant in Pain Management
and Anaesthesia, 6 Dales Way,
Tranmere Park, Guiseley,
Leeds, UK

Dr Louise Lynch*
D ward, Seacroft Hospital, York
Road, Leeds, UK

**Dr Rajesh Menon MD,
DipNb, FCARCSI**
Specialty Registrar, St James's
University Hospital,
Beckett Street, Leeds, UK

Dr Iordan Roussev Mihaylov
Specialist Trainee, Warwickshire
School of Anaesthesia, University
Hospitals Coventry and Warwick-
shire NHS Trust, Coventry, UK

Dr Rajesh Munglani
Consultant in Pain Medicine, West
Suffolk Hospital, Hardwick Lane,
Bury St Edmunds, UK

Sherdil Nath
Östra Esplanaden 6, 903 30 Umeå,
Sweden

Professor Jon H. Raphael
Graduate School, Ravensbury
House, Faculty of Health,
Westbourne Road, Edgbaston,
Birmingham City University, UK

**Dr Robert D. Searle FRCA
FFPMRCA**
Consultant in Anaesthesia and
Pain Management, The Pain Clinic,
Royal Cornwall Hospitals NHS
Trust, Truro, Cornwall, UK

Dr Manohar Lal Sharma
The Walton Centre for
Neurology and Neurosurgery
NHS Foundation Trust,
Lower lane, Liverpool, UK

**Dr Karim Nader
Shoukrey FRCA**
Specialist Registrar in Anaesthesia
and Pain Medicine, Addenbrooke's
Hospital, Cambridge University
Hospitals NHS Foundation Trust,
Hills Road, Cambridge, UK

Dr Karen Simpson
Consultant in Pain Medicine,
Leeds Teaching Hospitals,
Leeds, UK

**Mr Priyank Sinha MBBS,
MRCS Ed**
Specialist Registrar Neurosurgery,
Leeds General Infirmary, Great
George Street, Leeds, UK
Visiting Research Fellow, Leeds
Institute of Molecular Medicine,
Leeds, UK

**Mr Jake Timothy MD
FRCS(SN)**
Consultant Neurosurgeon,
Department of Neurosurgery,
Leeds General Infirmary,
Great George Street, Leeds, UK

Dr Peter Toomey
York Hospital, York, UK

Dr Simon Tordoff
Consultant in Anaesthesia and
Pain Management, University
Hospitals of Leicester NHS Trust,
Leicester General Hospital,
Gwendolen Road, Leicester, UK

Dr Thanthullu Vasu
Consultant in Anaesthetics
and Pain, Bangor,
North Wales, UK

*Has received honoraria from both Medtronic and Codman (Johnson & Johnson) and sat on an advisory board for Medtronic.

Symbols and abbreviations

📖	cross-reference
~	approximately
>	greater than
<	less than
AOL	aorta on left
AP	anteroposterior
ASA	American Society of Anesthesiologists
BMA	British Medical Association
BMD	bone mineral density
BMI	body mass index
CGRP	calcitonin-gene-related peptide
CN	cranial nerve
CNMP	chronic non-malignant pain
CO_2	carbon dioxide
COX	cyclo-oxygenase
CP	cancer-related pain
CPB	coeliac plexus block
CRPS	complex regional pain syndrome
CSF	cerebrospinal fluid
CT	computed tomography
Da	dalton(s)
DEXA	dual-energy X-ray absorptiometry
EMEA	European Medicines Evaluation Agency
ESRA	European Society of Regional Anaesthesia
EUS	enndoscopic-guided ultrasound
FBSS	failed back surgery syndrome
FDA	Food and Drug Administration
GABA	γ-aminobutyric acid
GMC	General Medical Council
GP	general practitioner
h	hour(s)
IDD	internal disc disruption
IPG	implanted pulse generator
ISIS	International Spine Intervention Society
IT	intrathecal
ITDD	intrathecal drug delivery

L	litre(s)
LA	local anaesthetic
LBP	lower back pain
LMWH	low molecular weight heparin
min	minute(s)
mL	millilitre(s)
MR	magnetic resonance
MRI	magnetic resonance imaging
MRSA	methicillin-resistant *Staphylococcus aureus*
NICE	National Institute for Health and Clinical Excellence
NMDA	*N*-methyl-D-aspartate
NSAID	non-steroidal anti-inflammatory drug
ODI	Oswestry Disability Index
PA	postero-anterior
PDD	percutaneous disc decompression
PDPH	post-dural puncture headache
psi	pounds per square inch
PSIS	posterior superior iliac spine
PTM	patient therapy manager
PVD	peripheral vascular disease
RA	refractory angina
RCR	Royal College of Radiologists
RF	radiofrequency
s	second(s)
SAP	superior articular process
SCS	spinal cord stimulation
SD	standard deviation
SIJ	sacroiliac joint
SNS	sacral nerve stimulation
SPECT	single-photon emission CT
SPG	sphenopalatine ganglion
SPGB	sphenopalatine ganglion block
STIR	short tau inversion recovery
$TcPO_2$	transcutaneous oxygen pressure
TENS	transcutaneous electrical nerve stimulation
USS	ultrasound scan/scanning
VAS	Visual Analogue Scale
WHO	World Health Organization

Applied anatomy and fluoroscopy for spinal interventions

S. Gupta and K. Dhandapani

Applied anatomy

Innervations of the cervical, thoracic, and lumbar facet joints

Facet joints are synovial joints formed by the inferior articular process of one vertebra and the superior articular process of the adjacent vertebra. The facet joints are innervated by the medial branches of the dorsal primary rami. The dorsal rami at each level supply branches to innervate the facet joint at the same level and the one below; this is fairly constant from C3 to C7/T1, T3/T4 to L4/L5. For example, to perform an L4/L5 facet joint block, the L3/L4 medial branches are blocked at L4/L5 (Fig. 1.1). However, at the cervical level, the medial branches are blocked at their respective levels. For example, to perform a C5/C6 facet joint block, the C5/C6 medial branches at C5/C6 are blocked (Fig. 1.2). The C2/C3 facet joint is innervated by the third occipital nerve. C3–C6 the medial branch is targeted from the centroid of the articular pillar. For a C7 medial branch block, the apex of the superior articular process is the target.

At the thoracic level the course of the medial branch is not consistent at all levels. The medial branch arises from the dorsal ramus within 5mm of the lateral margin of the intervertebral foramen and passes laterally. Opposite the tip of the transverse process of the vertebral body the medial branches curves dorsally, aiming for the lateral end of the superior border of the transverse process. This is consistent from T1 to T3 and at T9/10. For T11/T12 medial branches the targets are similar to those for lumbar medial branches. Between T4–T8 the medial branches do not always contact the transverse process and they may be suspended in the middle of the intertransverse space.

At the lumbar level the median branches are targeted slightly below the junction of the transverse process and the superior articular process. The L5/S1 joint is innervated by the L4 medial branch and the dorsal rami of L5. The dorsal ramus of L5 is approached at the groove formed by the ala of the sacrum and the superior articular process of S1.

Nerve supply of the intervertebral disc

Each intervertebral disc is composed of the outer annulus and the inner nucleus pulposus. In healthy adults, the outer third of the annulus is innervated; the inner annulus and the nucleus pulposus have no innervation. The posterior part of the disc is mainly supplied by sinuvertebral nerves that arise from the ventral primary ramus and ramus communicans. The posterior annulus also receives direct branches from the ventral primary ramus or ramus communicans. The lateral surfaces of the intervertebral discs are innervated by branches from the ventral primary rami and the rami communicantes (Fig. 1.3). The anterior part of the disc is innervated by the plexus formed around the anterior longitudinal ligament by rami communicantes or sympathetic nerves. In pathological intervertebral discs, growth of nerve fibres along granulation tissue can extend into the annulus and nucleus pulposus.

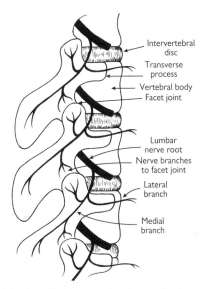

Fig. 1.1 Medial and lateral branches seen arising from the dorsal ramus. Facet joint articular branches seen arising from the medial branch.

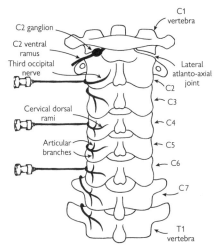

Fig. 1.2 Articular branches seen arising from the medial branches. On the left the needle tips are seen to block the third occipital nerve, C4 and C6 medial branches as seen in the AP view of the cervical spine.

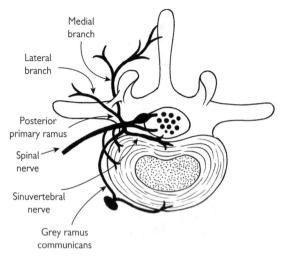

Fig. 1.3 Nerve supply to the lumbar intervertebral disc.

Innervation of the sacroiliac joint (SIJ)

The SIJ has an anterior and posterior joint line. The dorsal innervation of the SIJ is the predominant innervation in humans. The posterior joint is supplied by branches of the L5 dorsal ramus and the plexus formed by the dorsal rami of S1–S4. The lateral branch nerves have been described as exiting the sacral foramen from the 2 o'clock to 6 o'clock positions on the right or the 6 o'clock to 10 o'clock positions on the left at S1–S3 (if the dorsal sacral foramen is viewed as a clock face). The SIJ can be blocked by injecting local anaesthetic into either the SIJ or its nerve supply.

Fluoroscopic anatomy of the spine

General considerations

Fluoroscopy facilitates targeted therapy. There is evidence that a significant number of epidural injections may not be correctly placed if fluoroscopy is not used.

It is recommended that radio-opaque contrast is used before injecting any medication when performing interventional spinal procedures. A non-ionic water-soluble contrast that contains iodine is most commonly used. Iodine-containing agents are not recommended for patients with altered renal function and high volumes should not be used in patients on metformin.

A radiolucent operating table can facilitate the procedure, improve safety, and reduce the time required to perform the procedure. For all procedures at the lumbar level it is important to decrease the lumbar lordosis by placing a pillow under the patient's abdomen if he/she is prone.

When performing fluoroscopic-assisted interventional procedures it is important to use appropriate terminology and to discuss this with the radiographer. Tilting the C-arm towards the patient's head or feet is cephalic tilt or caudal tilt, respectively. Rotating the C-arm to the right or left side of the patient to obtain oblique views is rotation to the right or left, respectively.

To perform the procedures safely a 3D approach is essential. The three Ds stand for Direction of the needle in anteroposterior (AP) or oblique view, Depth of the needle in lateral view, and again Direction of the needle in AP or oblique view (Fig. 1.4).

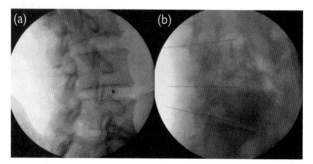

Fig. 1.4 (a) Direction of the needle is judged in the AP or oblique view. (b) Depth of the needle is judged in the lateral view.

Fluoroscopic anatomy of the lumbar spine

Obtain a clear AP view. In a true AP view the spinous process of the vertebra is in the centre with the pedicles on either side. After aligning the endplates of the vertebral bodies by cephalic or caudal tilt, the C-arm is rotated to the right or left to obtain a 'Scotty dog' view. Correct interpretation of key landmarks in AP, lateral, and oblique views is extremely important for safe fluoroscopic-assisted interventional procedures. The vertebral bodies, pedicles, laminae, transverse processes, spinous processes, superior articular processes, inferior articular processes, and pars intra-articularis should be identified on fluoroscopy as shown in Fig. 1.5.

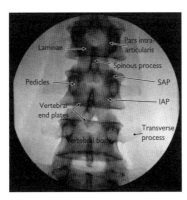

Fig. 1.5 The bony anatomy of the lumbar spine in the AP view. SAP, superior articular process; IAP, inferior articular process.

Identifying the superior articular process is the key when performing facet joint injections, medial branch blocks, discography, and therapeutic disc procedures. The pedicle is the key when performing nerve sleeve root injection, transforaminal epidural injection, or vertebroplasty. For nerve sleeve root injection the needle should be under the pedicle and just lateral to 6 o' clock position of the pedicle in AP view to avoid injecting into the dural sleeve or subarachnoid space. Target points are shown in Fig. 1.6.

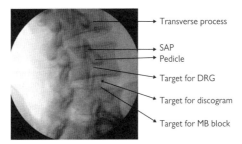

Fig. 1.6 Target points for various procedures. SAP, superior articular process; DRG, dorsal root ganglion; MB, medial branch.

After obtaining appropriate fluoroscopic images, the needle is directed to the target site under fluoroscopy using the 3D principle as already described. About 0.3–0.5 ml contrast is injected in AP view via low-volume tubing connected to the needle under continuous fluoroscopy. This is to confirm correct needle placement and rule out vascular spread before injecting any medication.

Fluoroscopic anatomy of sacroiliac joint

In the AP fluoroscopic image the posterior joint lines are medial and the anterior joint lines are lateral in most patients (Fig. 1.7(a)). SIJ injection can be done either by separating the anterior and posterior joint lines or by superimposing them (Fig. 1.7(b)). It is important to confirm under continuous fluoroscopy that the tip of the needle remains in the joint line before injecting contrast. On continuous fluoroscopy, if the tip of the needle appears to be displaced onto the bone it may not truly be in the joint space. In this situation another needle could be placed at the new joint line identified before injecting any contrast, as once contrast is injected it will be difficult to place a further needle. Inject the drug only after contrast confirmation.

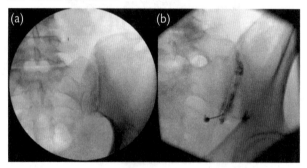

Fig. 1.7 (a) AP view of the SIJ: the medial joint line is the posterior joint line. (b) The posterior and anterior SI joint lines are aligned by contralateral oblique rotation. (Reproduced from Gupta S, Richardson J (2009). *Sacroiliac Joint Block.* In: *Interventional Pain Management: A Practical Approach.* Eds. Baneti, Bakshi, Gupta, Gehdoo, Figures 27.1 and 27.2, with permission from Jaypee Brothers Medical Publishers.)

Fluoroscopic anatomy of the cervical spine

In the cervical spine procedures can be performed with the patient in the lateral, supine, or prone positions. Cervical procedures are very risky and the key is to identify bony structures and landmarks. The 3D principle is used to navigate the needle to the target point. The vertebral levels can be counted down from C2 which has the largest articular process. Alternatively, levels can be counted up from C7, as the C7 transverse process slants downwards and the T1 transverse process is directed upwards.

For medial branch block a true lateral view that superimposes the right and left articular process is obtained with no parallax (Figs. 1.8(a) and 1.8(b)). The needle is directed to the centre of the rhomboid formed by joining the corners of the relevant pillar. In a patient with a short neck it can be difficult to visualize the C6 and/or C7 articular pillar, and it may be advisable to perform the procedure by obtaining an AP view with the patient prone (Fig. 1.8(c)).

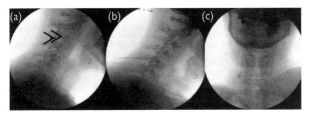

Fig. 1.8 (a) Lateral view of the cervical spine with parallax best seen at the C3 level (arrows). (b) The parallax seen in (a) has been eliminated by oblique rotation and tilt under continuous fluoroscopy; with the needle in position for C5 median branch block or radiofrequency neurotomy. (c) AP view showing the downward slanting transverse process of C7. The needle is in position for C7 medial branch block.

Fluoroscopic anatomy of the thoracic spine

It is difficult to identify the bony anatomy of the thoracic spine because of the ribs. Obtain an AP view. Square the vertebral body endplate closest to the target entry point by cephalic or caudal tilt; identify the bony structures (Fig. 1.9(a)). Then obtain a right or left oblique view; identify the different structures of the thoracic vertebra depending on the procedure being performed. Use the 3D principle when advancing the needle. In the lateral view it can be difficult to identify the bony anatomical structures and swivel movements of the C-arm (wig-wag movements) to square the vertebral endplates can help to identify the intervertebral foramen and surrounding structures (Fig. 1.9(b)).

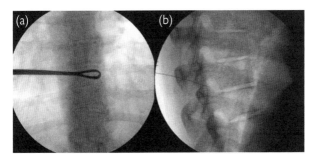

Fig. 1.9 (a) AP view of the thoracic spine with vertebral endplates squared off by caudal or cephalic tilt. (b) Lateral view of the thoracic spine with the vertebral endplates squared off by swivel movements of the C-arm (wig-wag movements).

Further reading

Bogduk N (1983). The innervation of the lumbar spine. *Spine* **8**: 286–93.

Bogduk N (2004) Cervical medial branch block. In: Bogduk N (ed.) *Practice Guidelines: Spinal Diagnositic and Treatment Procedures*. San Francisco, CA: International Spinal Intervention Society.

Bogduk N, Tynan W, Wilson AS (1981). The nerve supply to the human lumbar intervertebral discs. *J Anat* **132**: 39–56.

Chua WH (1994). *Clinical Anatomy of the Thoracic Dorsal Rami*. BMedSci Thesis, University of Newcastle, Australia.

Chua WH, Bogduk N (1995). The surgical anatomy of thoracic facet denervation. *Acta Neurochir* **136**: 140–4.

Fredman B, Nun MB, Zohar E, *et al.* (1999). Epidural steroids for treating 'failed back surgery syndrome'. Is fluoroscopy really necessary? *Anesth Analg* **88**: 367–72.

Groen G, Baljet B, Drukker J (1990). Nerves and nerve plexuses of the human vertebral columns. *Am J Anat*; **188**: 282–96.

Yin W, Willard F, Carreiro J, *et al.* (2003). Sensory stimulation-guided sacroiliac joint radio-frequency neurotomy. *Spine* **20**: 2419–25.

Chapter 2

Imaging in pain medicine

C. Groves and M. Chandramohan

Imaging modalities

Aims
- To understand the role of imaging in pain medicine.
- To know the advantages and limitations of each imaging modality.
- To be able to decide what imaging to choose and when to choose it.

Imaging modalities
- X-ray
- Ultrasound
- Fluoroscopy
- Isotope study
- Computed tomography (CT) scan
- Magnetic resonance imaging (MRI).

X-ray
- There is no specific role for plain X-ray in pain medicine.
- One of the most common radiological investigations requested by general practitioners (GPs) for patients presenting with back pain or joint pain.
- Can be useful to confirm the presence of degenerative disease and to exclude other causes of back or joint pain such as osteoporotic spinal fractures, inflammatory spondyloarthropathy, infection, and malignancy.

Ultrasound
- Used to confirm the clinical diagnosis of bursitis (subacromial bursitis, trochanteric bursitis, intermetatarsal bursitis) and to exclude conditions that can simulate bursitis such as shoulder rotator cuff tears.
- Used to guide an injection, particularly when conservative treatment fails or when the patient does not respond to unguided injections.
- Injection techniques:
  - injection of steroid and local anaesthetic (LA) for bursitis (sub-acromial, trochanteric, and intermetatarsal), paratenonitis, tenosynovitis, impingement syndromes, and Morton's neuroma
  - dry needling of refractory tendinosis (patellar tendinosis, plantar fasciitis, tennis elbow) with or without autologous blood injection
  - barbotage and percutaneous aspiration of calcific tendinosis.

Fluoroscopy
- Widely used by pain specialists to guide spinal interventions such as nerve root blocks, epidural injections, facet interventions, sacroiliac joint injections, nucleoplasty/nucleotomy, neurolysis, and vertebroplasty.
- Peripheral joint injections (shoulder, acromioclavicular joint, sternoclavicular joint, elbow, wrist, hip, knee, ankle, and small joints of hand and foot) are usually performed by musculoskeletal radiologists.

Isotope scan
- No specific role in pain medicine.
- Can be useful to exclude metastasis as a cause of back pain in patients with known malignancy, particularly when MRI is contraindicated.
- Sensitive but not specific to distinguish osteoporotic vertebral fracture from malignant vertebral collapse reliably, particularly when vertebroplasty is contemplated.

Computed tomography (CT)
- Exquisite bone detail—e.g. to confirm pars interarticularis defects in lytic spondylolysthesis (Fig. 2.1).
- Image acquisition is rapid, requiring seconds rather than the approximately 30 minutes needed for MRI. This may be helpful for patients who find MRI difficult to tolerate.
- Can demonstrate disc bulges (Fig. 2.2) and spinal stenosis. It is useful for claustrophobics who cannot tolerate MRI and for patients with spinal cord stimulators in whom MRI is contraindicated.

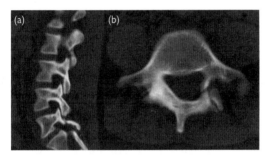

Fig. 2.1 (a) CT scan lumbar spine sagittal reformat showing spondylolysis of L5 on the left. (b) CT scan lumbar spine axial image of the same patient showing spondylolysis of L5 on the left.

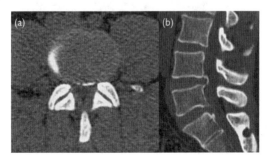

Fig. 2.2 (a) CT scan lumbar spine axial image showing a calcified annular disc bulge at L4/L5. (b) CT scan lumbar spine sagittal reformat of the same patient showing a calcified disc bulge at L4/L5.

- Has multiplanar capability, allowing abnormalities to be assessed in three planes. This is particularly helpful in trauma.
- Assesses complex congenital spines for hemi-vertebrae/fusion defects.
- Helpful for preoperative assessment for vertebroplasty to confirm an intact posterior vertebral body wall and pedicles.
- Image-guided interventions such as bone biopsy or epidural nerve root injection can be performed using CT. This is not the case for MRI.

Limitations of CT

- High radiation penalty. It depends on the scanner used, but a CT scan is equivalent to ~400 chest radiographs.
- Does not provide assessment of the cord.
- Intraspinal haemorrhage or tumour may not be apparent.
- Limited information about the disc—e.g. disc dehydration and annular fissures. The latter are not shown with CT.

Magnetic resonance imaging (MR or MRI)

- Used for cord and nerve root assessment.
- Provides information about the discs, and is able to demonstrate disc dehydration, annular fissures, and herniation (Fig. 2.3).
- Vertebral endplates are well demonstrated, and the use of contrast allows degenerative endplate changes to be distinguished from early discitis (Fig. 2.4).
- Ligament disruption can be excluded with MRI. This is important in trauma.
- MRI is the modality of choice to evaluate intraspinal tumours, haemorrhage, and intraspinal abscess.
- Useful for the assessment of the postoperative spine; epidural fibrosis can be confirmed with contrast-enhanced MRI (Fig. 2.5).
- Can be used for bone marrow pathology. May be able to distinguish between a pathological and an osteoporotic fracture in the spine.
- Sensitive to bone marrow oedema and sclerosis (Fig. 2.6). Can help to age vertebral fractures. It can also be used to assess activity of sacroilieitis.

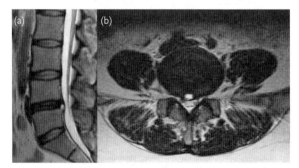

Fig. 2.3 (a) MRI sagittal T_2-weighted sequence showing an annular fissure in the degenerative L4/L5 disc. (b) Axial T_2-weighted sequence of the same patient demonstrating posterior annular fissure.

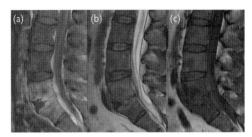

Fig. 2.4 (a) Post-gadolinium T$_1$-weighted image showing a non-enhancing abscess in the L5/S1 disc anteriorly, differentiating discitis from Modic type 1 changes. (b) Sagittal T$_2$-weighted sequence of the same patient showing oedema of the vertebral endplates of L5/S1 due to discitis. (c) Sagittal T$_1$-weighted sequence demonstrating loss of L5/S1 disc height with destruction of the endplates consistent with discitis.

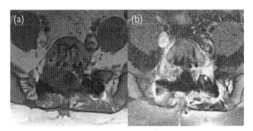

Fig. 2.5 (a) Axial T$_1$-weighted image of a postoperative spine at L5/S1 showing right sided soft tissue mass consistent with epidural fibrosis. (b) Post-contrast axial T$_1$-weighted image of the same patient showing heterogeneous enhancement of the epidural soft tissue mass consistent with epidural fibrosis.

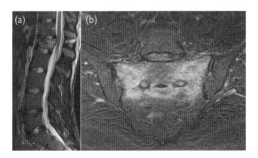

Fig. 2.6 (a) Sagittal short T$_1$ inversion recovery (STIR) sequence of a young gymnast showing oedema of the L1 vertebral body due to acute burst fracture. (b) Coronal STIR sequence of an elderly female patient showing extensive oedema of the sacrum due to a sacral insufficiency fracture.

Limitations of MRI

- Currently takes 20–40min to acquire a full series for a spinal study.
- The patient must be able to keep still, otherwise the images are blurred.
- Most MRI scanners in use are closed bore, and there is a significant failure rate due to claustrophobia.
- Spinal abnormality is very common in the older patient. MRI findings are only significant if they fit the clinical picture.
- There are some absolute and many relative contraindications to MRI.
  - Absolute contraindications: cardiac pacemaker, metal fragments in the eye, spinal cord stimulator.
  - Relative contraindications: certain ventriculoperitoneal shunts; certain heart valves.

The list of relative contraindications is long and depends on the magnet strength, the type of device, and the manufacturer. If the referrer has any doubt, they should discuss the case with their MR radiographers. The MR compatibility of most devices can also be checked on the website www.mrisafety.com.

Disc disease and back pain

Disc disease

- The spinal disc consists of a central nucleus pulposus encased within the tough outer ring of the annulus fibrosus.
- As the disc ages, the nucleus pulposus begins to dry out and the MR signal changes. Radiologists may comment on 'disc dehydration'.
- The aging annulus fibrosus is prone to tear, particularly at its posterior margin, producing annular fissures. These are seen as 'high-intensity zones' within the annulus with MRI (Fig. 2.7) and are thought to be painful.
- An annular fissure (also called an annular tear or high-intensity zone) is a rim rent in the annulus fibrosus, which may allow disc material from the nucleus pulposus to extrude into the spinal canal.
- Annular fissures can tear completely, allowing the nucleus pulposus to extrude into the central canal where it may remain contained by the posterior longitudinal ligament. Disc material which escapes into the epidural space and separates completely from its parent disc is said to be sequestrated (Fig. 2.8).
- Degenerative changes also involve the vertebral endplates. There are three recognized phases of degenerative endplate disease, termed Modic types 1, 2, and 3.
- Modic type 1 is the earliest phase where the endplates become oedematous (Fig. 2.9). They initially heal with fatty deposition (Modic type 2), and finally fibrose (Modic type 3). These phases are well shown with MRI.

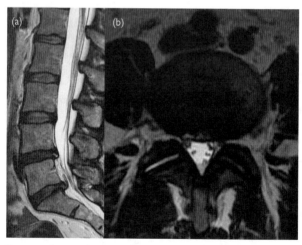

Fig. 2.7 (a) Sagittal T_2-weighted image demonstrating an annular fissure of the degenerative L4/L5 and L5S1 discs. (b) Axial T_2-weighted image of the same patient showing a posterior annular tear or fissure.

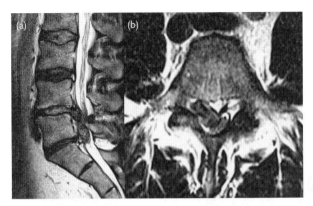

Fig. 2.8 (a) MRI T_2-weighted sequence sagittal image showing sequestrated disc material from the L4/L5 disc in the spinal canal. (b) Axial T_2-weighted image of the same patient showing sequestrated disc material in the spinal canal.

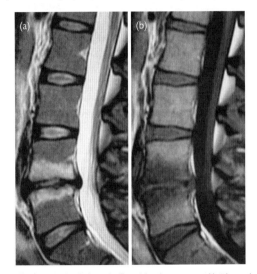

Fig. 2.9 Oedema appears dark on the T_1-weighted sequence and bright on the T_2-weighted sequence. (a) Sagittal T_1-weighted sequence of the lumbar spine showing oedema of the vertebral endplates of L4/L5 consistent with Modic type 1 changes. (b) Sagittal T_2-weighted sequence of the same patient showing high-signal oedema of the L4/L5 vertebral endplates in Modic type 1 changes.

Radiologist's description of disc lesions

There are many methods for naming disc disease in the literature, with no universally agreed nomenclature. We present the system used at our institution.

- The term 'disc bulge' is used in preference to disc herniation for broad-based disc prolapse.
- A 'focal' disc bulge (protrusion and extrusion) is described by its position in the canal: central, right, or left paracentral, or far lateral where the disc extends into the paraspinal region (Fig. 2.10).
- Disc material extrusions (nucleus pulposus squeezed through torn annulus fibrosus) are described as 'contained' if they are constrained by the posterior longitudinal ligament, and 'sequestrated' if they are separated from their parent discs.

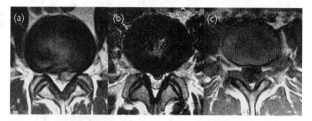

Fig. 2.10 Axial T_2-weighted images of (a) left paracentral disc protrusion and (b) posterior and central disc protrusion. (c) Axial T_1-weighted image of left far-lateral disc protrusion.

Spinal stenosis

- Narrowing of the passages of the spinal canal resulting in nerve compression.
- Usually caused by a combination of disc herniation, facet hypertrophy, and buckling of the ligamentum flavum.
- Three types:
  - central canal stenosis
  - lateral recess stenosis
  - exit foraminal stenosis (Fig. 2.11).
- Spinal stenosis results from degenerative changes and it is often multilevel. It is usually found in the lumbar spine. Symptoms are commonly due to a combination of all three types of spinal stenosis
- Spinal stenosis can be graded as mild, moderate, or severe. There is no universally agreed grading system in the literature, and currently grading is subjective
- At our institution, mild spinal stenosis is suggested when the central canal is narrowed with respect to the levels above and below. Moderate central canal stenosis results in crowding of the nerve roots. Severe spinal stenosis results in almost complete obliteration of the central canal and buckling of the more proximal cauda equina.

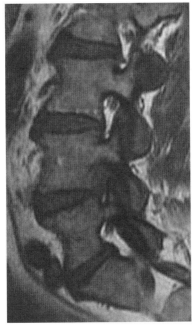

Fig. 2.11 Sagittal MR image showing severe L4/L5 exit foraminal stenosis due to foraminal disc protrusion.

Making the best use of your radiologist

- The radiologist is completely reliant on the clinical information that you provide, so it must be comprehensive and legible.
- Make use of the 'differential diagnosis' box on the request form. This tells the radiologist what conditions you would like to exclude.
- If you are not sure which test is appropriate, contact the radiologist who will be happy to discuss options.
- If you need to exclude urgent conditions, such as cord compression, epidural abscess, haematoma, or discitis, it is crucial to speak to the radiologist who is usually able to ensure that the necessary imaging is done in a timely manner.
- Spinal abnormalities are common in older patients, but they are only significant if the patient's history and examination correlate with the imaging findings.

Imaging protocol for back pain
- X-ray:
  - suspected spondylolisthesis or ankylosing spondylitis in a young patient.
- MRI:
  - progressive neurology
  - discogenic low back pain.
- CT or CT myelography:
  - MRI contraindicated
  - MRI equivocal.
- Problem solving tools:
  - diagnostic injections
  - discography.

Further reading

Fritz J, Niemeyer T, Clasen S, et al. (2007). Management of chronic low back pain: rationales, principles, and targets of imaging-guided spinal injections. *Radiographics* **27**: 1751–71.

RCR (2007). *Making the Best Use of Clinical Radiology Services (MBUR)* (6th edn). London: Royal College of Radiologists.

Sheehan NJ (2010). Magnetic resonance imaging for low back pain: indications and limitations. *Ann Rheum Dis* **69**: 7–11.

Drugs, equipment, and basic principles of spinal interventions

R. Mihaylov, S. Balasubramanian, and T. Vasu

Basic principles

Introduction

Spinal interventional injections have an important role in the multimodal management of patients suffering with persistent pain when appropriately selected and performed. They are used for either precision diagnosis or therapeutic purposes.

Patient selection

Selection of patients on the basis of careful history and complete physical examination is vital for the success of any interventional procedure. Although diagnostic imaging studies have limitations in identifying the precise source of pain, they may be needed prior to procedures such as nerve root blocks. All 'red flags' should be considered in the differential diagnosis before selecting a patient for intervention. These procedures should be part of a multidisciplinary care programme aimed at reduction in pain and improvement in physical function.

Contraindications

Absolute

- Patient is unable or unwilling to consent to the procedure
- Patient is unable to cooperate during the procedure
- Localized infection at the needle entry site
- Abnormal clotting (due to drugs or disease) for neuraxial blocks (e.g. epidural injections).

Relative

- Allergy to drugs used in the procedure (including contrast agents)
- Distorted anatomy
- Systemic infection
- Significant immunocompromise
- Pregnancy (may preclude use of fluoroscopy—ultrasound-guided blocks possible)
- Abnormal clotting (due to drugs or diseases) for paraxial blocks (e.g. facet injections)
- Unstable neurological disease.

Anticoagulants

No guidelines exist for the management of anticoagulated patients considered for interventional pain procedures. The European Society of Regional Anaesthesia (ESRA) recommendations for neuraxial blocks in the presence of anticoagulants are summarized in Table 3.1.

Therapeutic anticoagulation is an absolute contraindication to all epidural injections. It is relatively contraindicated for sacroiliac and zygoapophyseal joint injections, necessitating a risk–benefit assessment.

There is controversy regarding the risks associated with non-steroidal anti-inflammatory drugs (NSAIDs). International Spine Intervention Society (ISIS) guidelines state that concurrent treatment with NSAIDs may need to be discontinued prior to the conduct of spinal injections. The practice of stopping NSAIDs for 4–7 days is particularly prevalent in the USA.

Table 3.1 ESRA guidelines for neuraxial procedures in anticoagulated patients

Anticoagulant	Recommendation
Antiplatelet agents	NSAIDS (including aspirin): no contraindication
	Clopidogrel: discontinue for 7 days prior to procedure
Warfarin	Discontinue for 4–5 days prior to procedure Target INR <1.4
Low molecular weight heparin (LMWH)	Thromboprophylactic dose: delay procedure for 12h after last dose
	Treatment dose: delay procedure for 24h after last dose
	LMWH should not be administered for at least 2–4h after the procedure

Data from ESRA recommendations.

Although the incidence of epidural haematomas is very low, so is the incidence of thromboembolic events following a brief period of normalization of coagulation in anticoagulated patients. Thorough risk–benefit evaluation together with adequate explanation and patient involvement in the decision-making process are vital in such cases.

The decision to interrupt any anticoagulant should be made with multidisciplinary involvement, including liaison with the cardiologist or general practitioner.

Consent

In the UK, written and signed consent should be obtained as mandated by General Medical Council (GMC) guidance. The consenting physician must provide sufficient patient-specific information including a description of the intended procedure, its rationale (diagnostic or therapeutic), alternative options, complications and their likelihood, and risks versus benefits. Infrequent but serious complications must be discussed. Patients should understand which of their symptoms are targeted by the intervention and if these are likely to recur. In the UK consent for patients who may lack capacity is governed by the Mental Capacity Act 2005 which came into force in 2007.

Patient information

Time pressures may occasionally limit clinicians' abilities to provide the optimal amount of information and support to their patients. According to GMC consent guidance, resources such as patient information leaflets, expert patient programmes, and support groups should be used. Some internet resources containing patient information are:

- http://www.britishpainsociety.org/pub_patient.htm
- http://www.paincoalition.org.uk
- http://www.handlepain.co.uk
- http://www.managepain.co.uk
- http://www.painclinic.org/informationleaflets.htm

Personnel and facilities

Medical personnel

The team should consist of at least an interventional pain specialist helped by a designated trained assistant, a radiographer, and nursing staff. The interventional pain specialist is responsible for staff supervision and overall patient care and safety. Clinical governance standards apply as in any other area of clinical work. Procedures for checking patient identity, site and nature of planned procedure, patient preparation, and readiness of equipment should meet the standards expected according to the World Health Organization (WHO) surgical safety checklist.

Procedure room

The procedure room should be spacious enough for the safe accommodation of the patient, the medical personnel, and the equipment. A full range of antiseptics must be available. A surgical handwash facility must be located in close proximity. There should be facilities for non-invasive blood pressure, pulse oximetry, and ECG monitoring. Full resuscitation facilities and equipment must be immediately available.

Radiological equipment

Use of fluoroscopy is mandatory for a variety of procedures including epidural, median branch, sympathetic, and sacroiliac joint blocks. This is confirmed by the position statement of ISIS, stating that fluoroscopic guidance is the only means by which precision and patient safety can be guaranteed for spinal injections. The C-arm fluoroscope which allows delivery of the X-ray beam at any angle is in universal use. The fluoroscope must be connected to a monitor capable of displaying and storing images.

Radiation protection equipment

The use of radiation gowns with minimum lead protection of 0.35mm is mandatory. Radiation gloves, thyroid shields, forearm shields, and leaded eye-protective glasses are also available. However, protection attire should not provide a false sense of security. It is essential to maintain a suitable distance from the intensifier, if appropriate and safe to do so. Other staff in the vicinity should be advised and educated appropriately. Pulsed fluoroscopy or single exposures, rather than continuous radiation, should be preferred whenever possible.

Ultrasound equipment

Ultrasound is an increasingly used imaging technique for spinal injections. Limitations of its use include the need to overcome a learning curve, inability to visualize contrast spread, and difficulty in interpreting images in the presence of distorted anatomy, such as previous back surgery. Benefits include portability, avoidance of radiation hazards, use of real-time imaging, safety during pregnancy, and cost savings in terms of staff and equipment. Ultrasound transducers generate different frequencies: low-frequency probes (2–5MHz) are used to image deeper structures, including lumbar epidurals and paravertebral injections, and high-frequency probes (5–10MHz) are used for superficial blocks such as caudal epidurals.

Procedural table

The tipping table must be radiolucent as fluoroscopy use is standard. It must be possible to image the whole spine including the L5/S1 disc.

Recovery facilities

Patients must recover in a specially designated post-anaesthesia care area staffed by trained personnel. Drugs, equipment, fluids, and protocols for resuscitation and management of complications should be immediately available. An emergency alert system must be in place.

Equipment

Spinal needles

Spinal needles with two types of bevel are used: cutting (sharp-tipped) and non-cutting (blunt-tipped). Common commercially available cutting needles include Quincke and Yale. These penetrate tissues with greater ease and are preferred by many practitioners. Popular non-cutting needles include Sprotte and Whitacre which have a lateral orifice proximal to their 'pencil-point' tip. The perceived advantage of non-cutting needles is reduced risk of damage to neural and vascular tissues. In the UK, 22G needles are commonly used for most spinal interventions.

Navigating the spinal needle

The bevel opening of the spinal needle correlates with the elevated mark on its hub, and the needle usually moves in the opposite direction to the bevel opening (Fig. 3.1). With experience, the interventionalist will become increasingly skilled at bevel control and adjustments of tension imparted on the needle, allowing its safe and correct placement. Bending the needle (along the direction of the bevel) may help navigation.

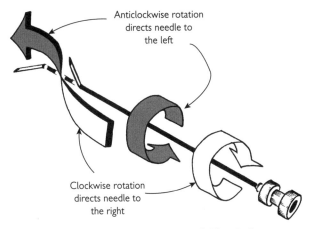

Anticlockwise rotation directs needle to the left

Clockwise rotation directs needle to the right

Fig. 3.1 Illustration explaining the magic of a bent needle. This aids effective navigation of the bent needle.

Epidural needles

The most common type of epidural needle used in the UK and worldwide is the Tuohy needle. It has a total length of 10cm, with the shaft being 8cm long. A 15cm Tuohy needle is available for obese patients. Two sizes are available: 16G and 18G. The bevel has a blunt design to minimize the risk of dural puncture and is curved at 20° relative to the shaft to enable catheter guidance. Epidural needles are used for interlaminar lumbar, thoracic, and cervical epidural injections. Regional block needles are commonly used to perform caudal epidural injections.

Radiofrequency (RF) needles

RF needles are fully electrically insulated except for their 5–10mm tip which conducts the RF current. The tissue temperature is constantly measured by a 27G thermocouple inserted through the 18G, 20G, or 22G RF needle. Thermal radiofrequency lesioning is achieved by maintaining a target temperature of 80–85°C for a period of 60–90s. The recommended protocol for pulsed RF as described in the ISIS position paper is the delivery of 50,000 Hz current at 20 ms pulses with frequency of 2 pulses per second. The temperature should be limited to less than 42 degrees C.

RF generators

RF generators produce an alternating current in the RF range (kHz) at the tip of the RF needle. A typical unit consists of a current generator, temperature monitor, timer, current and voltage monitor, and tissue impedance monitor. A built-in nerve stimulator allows sensory testing (50 or 100Hz) and motor testing (1–2Hz).

Pharmacology

Local anaesthetics

LAs are used for diagnostic and therapeutic interventions. They may act therapeutically by breaking the pain–spasm–pain cycle.

Mechanism of action

LAs bind to specific intracellular sites within voltage-gated sodium channels of neuronal tissues, thereby blocking the influx of sodium ions during membrane depolarization. Generation and propagation of action potentials are reversibly blocked.

Common LA formulations

Lidocaine hydrochloride

Lidocaine has a fast onset and short duration of action. It is used in a variety of concentrations (0.5–4%). At higher concentrations lidocaine produces a dense motor block. Lidocaine 1% or 2% is used for skin and subcutaneous infiltration. Adequate infiltration can gain the patient's confidence, thus avoiding the need for sedation.

Bupivacaine hydrochloride

Bupivacaine has a medium onset and a long duration of action, with the block lasting up to several hours. It is used in concentrations ranging from 0.1% to 0.5%. Bupivacaine is more cardiotoxic than equipotent lidocaine doses.

Levobupivacaine

Levobupivacaine is an S-enantiomer of bupivacaine that is approximately 10% less potent than racemic bupivacaine. Its main advantage over the racemic preparation is reduced cardiac toxicity.

LA toxicity

Toxicity depends on LA potency, site of injection, rate of plasma concentration rise, amount injected, and protein binding. Inadvertent intra-vascular injection of a subtoxic dose may produce toxicity due to a rapid rise in plasma concentration. Administration of LAs via the caudal and epidural routes is associated with significant systemic uptake.

The *British National Formulary* gives the following maximum safe doses for LAs when they are delivered via the lumbar epidural route in a fit adult of average size: lidocaine 200mg; bupivacaine 100mg; levo-bupivacaine 150mg; ropivacaine 200mg.

The Association of Anaesthetists of Great Britain and Northern Ireland has produced guidelines for the management of severe LA toxicity. A recent development has been the use of intravenous lipid emulsion, which should be available in all areas where LAs are used.

Steroids

Mechanism of action

Steroids are thought to act by inhibition of proinflammatory mediator production, exertion of a membrane-stabilizing effect, and suppression of dorsal horn neuronal sensitization.

Common steroid formulations

Commonly used injectable steroids include methylprednisolone acetate (Depo-Medrol), triamcinolone (Aristocort, Kenalog), and dexamethasone. These steroid formulations contain a number of other chemicals and buffers, including benzyl alcohol in Depo-Medrol, Aristocort and Kenalog, and polyethylene glycol in Depo-Medrol and Aristocort.

There is insufficient evidence about the relative efficacy, safety, optimal dose, and frequency of different steroid preparations. Commonly used doses are 20–80mg for methylprednisolone and triamcinolone, and 2–8mg for dexamethasone. There seems to be no significant difference in analgesic efficacy when comparing 40mg with 80mg doses of methyl-prednisolone.

Systemic complications

The risk of systemic complications related to epidural steroids appears to be small. Rare case reports have described short-term adrenal suppression, development of transient secondary Cushing's syndrome, and development of bone demineralization associated with increased risk of fractures. Steroids can impair glycaemic control; at-risk patients such as diabetics must be informed of this effect.

Particulate steroids

Case reports have implicated epidural injections of methylprednisolone and triamcinolone in causing serious injuries to the spinal cord and brain. A proposed mechanism of injury is vascular embolization of steroid particles and aggregates after iatrogenic intra-arterial injection. No such complications have been reported with dexamethasone, a non-particulate steroid with diameter ~0.5µm. Dexamethasone is now preferred by many pain specialists for use in cervical transforaminal epidurals.

Epidurally injected steroids

Currently there is no evidence of any steroid-related deleterious effects following steroidal deposition in the epidural space.

Both interlaminar and transforaminal epidural steroid injections carry the risk of iatrogenic spinal cord injury. There has been concern that the transforaminal approach, especially at cervical level, is associated with greater risks of adverse events than the interlaminar route. This may be due to inadvertent injections into the vertebral or radicular arteries at cervical level and the artery of Adamciewicz at the lumbar and thoracic levels.

Intrathecal steroids

Accidental intrathecal injections of steroids carry a potential risk of neurotoxicity. In animal studies, supraclinical concentrations of poly-ethylene glycol reversibly altered nerve conduction characteristics. Reports have implicated benzyl alcohol in neuronal degeneration and paraplegia. Clinicians should be meticulous in minimizing the potential risk of inadvertent intrathecal steroid placement.

Volume and rate of epidural injections

Rapid administration of large-volume epidural injections is associated with significant adverse events, including retinal and cerebral haemorrhage. These risks increase with cervical-level injections and the presence of age-related degenerative changes such as spinal central canal or foraminal stenosis.

Precision targeting

Specific steroid epidural injections can be successfully delivered via the transforaminal route or catheter-guided interlaminar route by using cautiously injected volumes of 2–3mL.

Chemical neurolytic agents

Chemical neurolysis is the intentional injury of specifically targeted nerves by chemical agents. Neurolytic therapy primarily affects cell axons rather than cell bodies, thus enabling nervous tissue regeneration. Neurolytic effects typically last for 3–6 months. The commonly used agents are ethyl alcohol and phenol; both produce non-selective neural destruction.

Ethyl alcohol is commonly used in 50–100% concentrations. It diffuses freely through tissues. It is painful on injection, necessitating prior LA administration. Phenol is used in concentrations of 3–12%. It diffuses poorly and this confers the advantage of highly localized spread. Phenol has LA properties, producing immediate analgesic effect following successful administration.

During intrathecal administration, ethyl alcohol is hypobaric with respect to cerebrospinal fluid (CSF). Hence patients must be positioned with the affected side uppermost and at a forward 45° tilt. Phenol is hyperbaric; thus the painful side must be placed in a dependent position.

Radio-opaque contrast agents

Radio-opaque contrast agents are used to locate needle position accurately, delineate anatomical structures, and visualize spread of contrast medium. The use of contrast is mandatory for all fluoroscopically guided epidural injections.

Non-ionic hydrophilic agents must be used for epidural injections becaise of their lower risk of neurotoxicity compared with ionic agents. Non-ionic agents have a lower osmolality, which further reduces the incidence of adverse effects. Commonly used non-ionic agents include the iodine-based agents iohexol (Omnipaque 150 or 300) and iopamidol (Isovue). Contrast agents used for spinal injections must be licensed for intrathecal use in case of inadvertent intrathecal injection.

Major adverse events include severe allergic reactions and nephro-toxicity.

Absolute contraindication to use of contrast agents is known allergy to iodine products. Relative contraindications include convulsive disorders, pre-existing renal disease, and dehydration.

Antiseptic agents

The use of antiseptic skin preparations is an essential antiseptic precaution. Commonly used agents include isopropyl alcohol, chlorhexidine gluconate, and povidone–iodine (Betadine).

Isopropyl alcohol

Isopropyl alcohol 70% acts by denaturing microbial proteins. It has a rapid onset and a wide spectrum of action. Alcohol demonstrates excellent antimicrobial activity but its effectiveness is limited by lack of any residual activity. It is highly flammable.

Povidone–iodine

Povidone–iodine acts by releasing free iodine which oxidizes microbial cytoplasmic and membrane proteins. It is commonly available in 2% spray and 10% ointment. Povidone–iodine has an intermediate speed of onset, a wide spectrum of action, and limited residual activity. Regular use should be avoided in patients with thyroid disorders or those on lithium therapy.

Chlorhexidine gluconate

Chlorhexidine acts by disrupting microbial cellular membranes and is commonly used in 0.5% and 2% concentrations. It has an intermediate speed of onset, a long duration, and a wide spectrum of action. Chlorhexidine demonstrates superior clinical efficacy to povidone–iodine in terms of antimicrobial effect and residual activity.

Chlorhexidine gluconate in 70% isopropyl alcohol formulations combine the benefits of a significant immediate antimicrobial effect with excellent residual activity. Chlorhexidine concentrations of 0.5% and 2% are available. The current consensus is that 0.5% chlorhexidine in 70% isopropyl alcohol is the skin antiseptic of choice for regional anaesthesia.

Reports have implicated the use of 2% chlorhexidine skin preparations with arachnoiditis following central neuraxial blocks. It is advised that chlorhexidine concentrations >0.5% should not be used prior to spinal and epidural injections.

Training and patient care

Training

Currently, undergraduate courses in medicine do not provide training in interventional pain procedures.

In the UK the Faculty of Pain Medicine of the Royal College of Anaesthetists has developed a curriculum, training programme, examination, and assessments for pain medicine. There has been an increase in the availability of workshops and courses that allow participants to observe and obtain 'hands-on' experience. Cadaver workshops may be helpful.

Nursing and allied health professionals

Recovery and theatre staff must be competent in basic life support provision, assessment of vital signs, assessment of overall patient status, management of conscious sedation, and patient positioning. All staff members who are in contact with patients should receive a checklist of general contraindications so that problems are identified and promptly communicated. Staff must also be educated on the principles of persistent pain management and the biopsychosocial model of pain.

Pre-procedure fasting

Pre-procedure fasting is mandatory for procedures requiring conscious sedation. However, the authors rarely use sedation. Fasting is indicated prior to epidural injections containing LAs, as there is a potential for subarachnoid spread. The authors advise pre-procedure fasting for all epidural injections, sympathetic blocks, procedures with a risk of pneumothorax, intra-abdominal blocks, and invasive cervical procedures. The fasting period is 6h for solids and 2h for clear fluids.

Peri-procedure monitoring

In the UK recommendations concerning the minimal standards of monitoring required for epidural injections have been published jointly by the British Pain Society and the Royal College of Anaesthetists. Heart rate, non-invasive blood pressure, and pulse oximetry are recommended during and after all procedures where LA is placed near the dural sac.

Monitoring is also required for interventions that may result in significant haemodynamic disturbances, such as coeliac or lumbar sympathetic plexus blocks, and for high-risk patients. These include patients with significant comorbid conditions, relevant allergies, and previous vasovagal episodes, and in cases of sedation.

Monitoring is not routinely indicated for procedures such as lumbar zygo-apophyseal joint medial branch blocks or sacroiliac joint injections.

Use of sedation

Most minimally invasive spinal intervention procedures can be performed without sedation. ISIS does not recommend its routine use. Conscious sedation is reserved for selected cases where comorbid conditions necessitate it.

Inappropriately administered heavy sedation can reduce the patient's ability to provide feedback when vital structures are unintentionally reached with a needle. This lack of feedback has been implicated in cases of serious nerve damage that have resulted in catastrophic sequelae.

Many practitioners believe that the use of sedation to facilitate diagnostic spinal injections may influence outcome measures. This remains an area of controversy.

If conscious sedation has to be used, fasting, monitoring and intra-venous access are mandatory.

General anaesthesia is not recommended for most spinal interventional procedures.

Intravenous access

ISIS practice guidelines recommend the presence of intravenous access for all procedures in which needles are placed near the dural sac and for patients with relevant comorbidities. There is debate as to whether intravenous access is necessary if a small amount of LA is injected epidurally, although the potential risk of intrathecal spread is present.

The authors recommend intravenous access for all epidural injections, and especially for high-risk patients such as those with previous vasovagal episodes, relevant allergies, and significant comorbidities.

Follow-up and post-procedural care

Any procedure involving deposition of LA near the dural sac mandates observation in a monitored recovery area for at least 30min.

When diagnostic procedures are performed, post-procedural evaluation should be undertaken to measure and document changes in pain scores and improvement in physical activity.

Patients must be provided with clear follow-up instructions. They must be warned about a possible temporary increase in pain due to needle trauma and advised that steroids usually take at least 24h to achieve full effect. Appropriate analgesia must be provided to cover this period.

Patients may require assistance with mobilization following LA motor block. They should be warned to avoid driving, single-handed child care, and lifting heavy objects.

Patients should be instructed to seek medical advice if they experience unexpected neurological symptoms or other relevant problems such as fever and malaise. A mechanism should be in place to assess and manage patients if adverse events such as infection, post-dural puncture headache, or neurological problems occur.

The patient's GP should be informed of the details of the intervention and follow-up must be arranged. Outcomes should be evaluated in terms of pain relief and other measures such as sleep, daily activities, return to work, health-care utilization, medication use, and quality of life.

Further reading

Association of Anaesthetists of Great Britain and Ireland (2006). *Consent for Anaesthesia.* http://www.aagbi.org/publications/guidelines/docs/consent06.pdf.

Association of Anaesthetists of Great Britain and Ireland (2010). *Management of Severe Local Anaesthetic Toxicity.* http://www.aagbi.org/publications/guidelines/docs/la_toxicity_2010.pdf.

Bogduk N (2004). Intravenous lines. In: *Practice Guidelines: Spinal Diagnostic and Treatment Procedures.* San Francisco, CA: ISIS.

Bogduk N (2004). On the use of sedations. In: *Practice Guidelines: Spinal Diagnostic and Treatment Procedures.* San Francisco, CA: ISIS.

Bogduk N (2006). ISIS position paper on pulsed radiofrequency. *Pain Med* **7**: 396–407.

European Society of Regional Anaesthesia and Pain Therapy (2007). *Regional Anaesthesia and Thromboembolism Prophylaxis/Anticoagulation.* http://www.esra-learning.com.

General Medical Council (2008). *Consent: Patients and Doctors Making Decisions Together.* http://www.gmc-uk.org/static/documents/content/Consent_2008.pdf.

International Spine Intervention Society (2006). *Position Statement on Fluoroscopic Guidance.* http://columbiapain.org/documents/FluoroscopicGuidance.pdf.

Prager JP, AprilI C (2009). Complications related to sedation and anesthesia for interventional pain therapies. *Pain Med* **19**: S121–7.

Royal College of Anaesthetists and the British Pain Society (2002). *Recommendations on the Use of Epidural Injections for the Treatment of Back Pain and Leg Pain of Spinal Origin.* http://www.rcoa.ac.uk/docs/epidural-injections.pdf.

Smith HS, Chopra H, Patel VB, Frey ME, Rastogi H (2009). Systematic review of the role of sedation in diagnostic spinal interventional techniques. *Pain Physician* **12**: 195–206.

WHO (2008). *Surgical Safety Checklist.* http://www.who.int/patientsafety/safesurgery/tools_resources/SSSL_Checklist_finalJun08.pdf.

Lumbar spine interventions

*G. Baranidharan, J.H. Raphael, R. Menon, S. Nath,
S. Gupta, and N. Evans*

Caudal epidural

Introduction

Caudal epidural steroid injections are favoured for patients with lumbar spinal pain for two reasons.
- They are easy and less painful to perform
- Most disc-related problems are at L5/S1 and L4/5, which can easily be accessed from the caudal route

The advantage of a caudal epidural is that the injectate also spreads to the anterior epidural space, which is where most of the inflammation occurs.

Anatomy

The caudal epidural space is the lowest portion of the epidural canal (Fig. 4.1). It can be entered through the sacral hiatus. The sacrum is a triangular bone consisting of five fused sacral vertebrae from S1 to S5. It articulates with the lumbar vertebrae at the cranial end and the coccyx at the caudal end. The sacral hiatus is a small defect at the lower part of the posterior wall of the sacrum which is formed by the failure of the laminae of S5/4 to meet and fuse in the mid-line. It can be felt at the bottom of the sacrum and is the ideal entry point into the caudal epidural space. The sacral canal contains the terminal parts of the dural sac ending between S1 and S3, the five sacral nerves, the coccygeal nerves (making up the cauda equina), the caudal epidural vessels, and fat.

Sacral hiatus

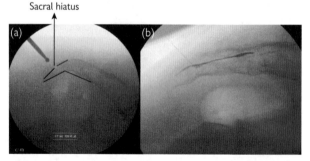

Fig. 4.1 (a) The caudal epidural space with the sacral hiatus clearly visible. (b) Contrast spread in the caudal space.

Indications

- Nerve root pain mainly secondary to disc prolapse at L5/S1 and possibly L4/5 (lumbar radiculopathy).
- Spinal stenosis at lower lumbar level.
- Post-laminectomy pain syndrome.
- Lower lumbar vertebral fractures.

- Pelvic pain in combination with sympathetic blocks, as the motor nerves for most of the pelvic innervation are around S1/2 especially in perineal pain.
- Pelvic, bladder, perineal, genital, rectal, scrotal and anal pain.
- Occasionally for conditions such as diabetic peripheral neuropathy, post-herpetic neuralgia, complex regional pain syndrome, and phantom limb pain.

Contraindications
- Systemic sepsis
- Bleeding diathesis
- Untreated infection.

Technique and position
Caudal epidural can be performed with patients in the prone or lateral position.

Prone position
The patient is positioned prone with a pillow under the abdomen.
- After aseptic preparation a lateral X-ray is taken to visualize the non-fusion of S4/5 (sacral hiatus).
- This is the entry point for a 22G needle. A distinct pop is felt as the needle enters the sacrococcygeal membrane. Once the needle is in place, a non-ionic contrast is injected. A caudal epidurogram is performed to make sure that the drug reaches the area of pathology.
- A Tuohy needle can also be used, and the needle can be directed to the side of the lesion.
- A combination of LA with steroid can be injected (7–10mL).
- Once the procedure is completed, the patient is placed flat on their back with the legs bent to reduce the lumbar lordosis, thus increasing the chances of the drug reaching the L5/S1 and L4/5 discs (the problem area in most lumbar radiculopathy).

Lateral position
The patient is placed in the lateral position and the same technique as for prone is used.

Fluoroscopy
The fluoroscopic view is normally a lateral view that gives a good indication of the sacral hiatus and helps to place the needle correctly. Once the needle is in place, an epidurogram is performed under continuous fluoroscopy in AP view. If there is significant inflammation and fibrosis, the dye may not reach the target site. A transforaminal epidural might be more useful in this situation.

Post-procedure care
The patient lies flat with legs bent for 10–15min. Routine observations are performed and the patient is warned about possible voiding difficulties.

Complications
- Epidural bleeding causing neurological sequelae.
- Infection.
- Nerve damage.
- The needle can also enter other areas (e.g. sub-periostium and bone marrow), with possible deposit of the drug outside the sacral canal causing pain for the first few weeks.
- Accidental intravascular injection, the risk of which can be reduced by continuous fluoroscopic epidurogram.

Tips

Needle entry does not need to be as far into the caudal epidural space as for a blind technique. The needle can be positioned at 90° in most patients. Once through the sacrococcygeal membrane, the drug does not come out of the membrane and a nice epidural spread should be seen. A Tuohy needle can be used, advancing it further cranially. The disadvantage of this is that it increases the risk of dural puncture and intrathecal placement of the LA and steroid.

Lumbar epidural

Introduction
Epidural steroid injections are placement of steroid with or without LA in the epidural space. Epidurals were traditionally performed using a blind approach without fluoroscopy. It is now recommended that fluoroscopy is used to increase the accuracy of placement of the needle into the epidural space and to deliver drugs to the appropriate level.

Anatomy of the epidural space
The epidural space runs from the foramen magnum to the sacrococcygeal membrane. It is bordered anteriorly by the posterior longitudinal ligaments and posteriorly by the vertebral laminae and ligamentum flavum. The lateral limits are formed by the vertebral pedicles and the intervertebral foramen. The lumbar epidural space lies at a depth of ~5–6mm at the level of L2/3 and contains epidural fat, veins, arteries, lymphatics, and connective tissue.

Indications
- Nerve root symptoms secondary to disc herniation
- Neuropathic leg symptoms related to spinal stenosis (spinal claudication)
- Discogenic back pain.

Epidurals have been used for differential neural blockade, but this is no longer extensively practised. Using this technique as a diagnostic block to look at a specific nerve root is inappropriate as the spread is to several nerve roots, even with a small amount of LA. Patients with radicular leg pain respond better to epidural injections.

Contraindications
- Patient refusal
- Untreated infection at the site or possibly systemic infection
- Bleeding diathesis/anticoagulants.

Relative contraindications
- Immunosuppression
- Anatomically difficult spine
- Allergy to radio-opaque conrast
- Lumbar spine surgery.

Technique and position
This procedure can be done in the sitting, lateral, or prone position.

Prone
- The patient is prone with a pillow under the abdomen to reduce lumbar lordosis and increase the interlaminar space.
- This is more comfortable for the patient and it is much easier to achieve an AP lateral view.

- Once the needle reaches the desired space, a lateral X-ray view should be obtained to confirm needle entry into the epidural space (just at the level of the lamina).
- Final confirmation is done by injecting non-ionic contrast. This will confirm the placement of the needle and likely spread of the contrast to the level being treated.

An 18G or 20G (Tuohy) epidural needle is available. The size of the needle will depend on the operator's choice. The smaller the needle, the less is the risk of post-dural puncture headache.

Sitting

The patient sits with a pillow on their knees to help arch the spine. Under aseptic conditions the level that requires injection is identified using an X-ray in the AP view followed by a lateral view to show the depth of the needle.

Loss of resistance to saline or air can be used depending on personal choice. Once the epidural space is identified, a non-ionic contrast is injected to visualize the spread (Fig. 4.2). This indicates whether the drug has reached the target area to be treated. If there is no appropriate spread (e.g. with a spinal stenosis at L3/4 and the drug spreading to L4/5 and L5/S1), alternative options such as a transforaminal route should be considered.

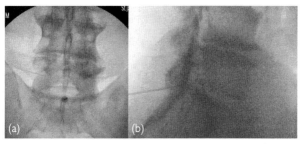

Fig. 4.2 (a) Needle in position to enter the L5/S1 epidural space. (b) Needle in positon and contrast spread in the epidural space.

Fluoroscopy

A true AP view is obtained at the level at which the epidural is to be performed. Cephalic or caudal tilt will square off the vertebral endplates. After the vertebral endplate closest to the target entry point is squared off, it should be possible to see the interlaminar space quite clearly. Ideally, the needle should be advanced either mid-line or slightly lateral depending on the indication for the epidural injection. If this is performed for single-level radicular pain, ideally the needle and bevel could be advanced slightly lateral as this facilitates the spread of the drug to the site of the pathology causing the patient's symptoms.

The injectate can be a combination of LA and steroid of volume 5–10mL, depending on the number of levels being treated. Studies show that a volume of about 2.5mL covers one vertebral level in the epidural space. It has also been suggested that toxic material is being washed off the nerve root. To increase the chances of this working; some operators use a larger volume of up to 20mL. There is no need to inject high volumes of LA, which is only acting as a carrier, as this increases the risk of total spinal and associated complications. The author uses 2mL of LA and 80mg triamcinalone diluted to the desired volume with normal saline (generally up to a total of 6 or 7mL). The steroid helps to decrease inflammation.

Post-procedure care

The patient should be monitored for at least 15–20min to check for inadvertent intrathecal administration of drug. If this happens, the patient will develop motor block depending upon the amount of LA used. There is also a risk of voiding difficulties, but this is unusual when the amount of LA used is negligible.

Complications

- Epidural bleeding causing neurological sequelae
- Infection
- Nerve damage
- Post-dural puncture headache.

The lumbar epidural space is highly vascular. intravenous placement can be recognized if there is bleeding back from the Tuohy needle or by epidurogram using fluoroscopy. Contrast being uptaken by venous drainage should prompt stopping injection of the drug.

Needle trauma related to epidural venous bleeding is generally self-limiting, but occasionally there can be uncontrolled bleeding leading to compression of the spinal cord.

Neurological complications can occur after a lumbar epidural, but this is very uncommon. If significant pain occurs during placement of an epidural, the operator should stop immediately and ascertain the cause of the pain to reduce the risk of neural trauma.

Failure

The level of the pathology is very important and the spread of contrast to the desired area helps to identify whether the epidural steroid injection will help the patient.

Tips

- Know your target disc and side before starting the procedure
- The pathology is in the anterior epidural space, and in the presence of a highly inflamed nerve root it is possible that the injectate may not reach the target site. In this case it might be better to use a transforaminal epidural if the epidurogram shows lack of spread to the desired nerve root
- Tight spinal stenosis might increase the chance of neurological complications. Viewing the MRI and choosing the entry level is very important in such patients.

Lumbar dorsal root blocks

Introduction

Lumbar dorsal nerve roots emerge from the spinal cord and pass laterally and inferiorly to join the corresponding ventral nerve roots to form the spinal nerves exiting from the spinal canal through the intervertebral foramina. The lumbar dorsal nerve roots transmit sensory information from corresponding dermatomes and sclerotomes that pass via synaptic connections to higher centres.

Lumbar dorsal nerve roots can be mechanically compressed and/or inflamed. This may manifest as lower-limb pain (radiculitis) and neurological abnormalities (e.g. sensory loss and motor weakness). Mechanical causes of dorsal root dysfunction include pressure or chemical irritation from prolapsed intervertebral discs, compression from facet joint hypertrophy, and narrowing of exit foramina as a result of osteoarthritis. Lumbar dorsal root blocks can be used diagnostically and/or therapeutically.

Diagnostic

It is possible to determine whether a particular nerve root is a significant source of symptoms by delivering LA to that nerve root only. However, the relationship between clinically observed dermatomes and the associated nerve roots is variable. Thus a dorsal root block can assist with the diagnosis of radicular pain and can also often define the pathological nerve root.

Therapeutic

It is common practice to administer steroids adjacent to a nerve root to provide analgesia arising from that particular nerve root that lasts longer than that provided by currently available LAs. Steroids have anti-inflammatory properties, and therefore if local inflammation is a significant part of the pathological and pain-producing process this strategy would be expected to reduce symptoms. Furthermore, steroids stabilize the electrical excitability of the cell membrane of C-fibres and so have a direct analgesic effect. When depot steroids are used, the dissolution of the agent from its site of injection is slow and may provide a longer-lasting therapeutic effect.

Evidence

There are no randomized controlled trials of diagnostic dorsal root blocks compared with placebo. Studies comparing the outcome of diagnostic blocks with findings at surgery suggest a high level of sensitivity (80–100%) and specificity (90%) for diagnosing pathology. There are several controlled trials of therapeutic dorsal root blocks, but the comparators, procedures, and follow-up periods differ. The results suggest that these injections provide relief better than placebo.

Patient selection

- Dermatomal distribution of neuropathic pain
- MRI and clinical correlation
- Failed conservative care.

It is important to have a reasonable target for the presumed pathology and painful symptoms—there should be a concordant history, supportive examination, and relevant investigations. Chronic pain often leads to psychosocial effects and these must be assessed. If a local target cannot confidently be assumed (e.g. if there is a widespread painful condition, significant pain behaviours, or psychological factors), targeted procedures are unlikely to be beneficial. In this situation non-interventional therapies may be needed. If a local target seems likely, one has to decide between pharmacological, physical, psychological, and interventional approaches, taking account the relative risks and benefits of each and the patient's preferences.

Contraindications

Absolute contraindications

- Infection at the site of injection
- Systemic infection
- Bleeding disorders
- Anticoagulants that cannot be stopped.

Relative contraindications

- Coexisting neurological conditions (the operator could be blamed for any subsequent deterioration)
- Cardiorespiratory disease which compromises function.

Procedure

The patient should be prone or lateral with the pathological side upper-most. Sedation may be necessary in some patients, but it is important to have an awake cooperative patient who is able to recognize inappropriate positioning of the needle; this may reduce the risk of nerve root injury. LA to the skin and subcutaneous tissues is valuable, and is better than relying on sedation.

Applied anatomy

The dorsal root typically passes inferolaterally from the spinal cord to exit the spinal canal through the intervertebral foramen. As a result there is a 'safe triangle' below the pedicle whose borders are the inferior border of the pedicle, a line running sagittally from its lateral border, and the dorsal root itself (Fig. 4.3). If a needle is sited in this area, this should reduce the chances of it entering the nerve root. The aim of the procedure is to deposit the therapeutic agent adjacent to the nerve root, not within it. In pathological circumstances, the nerve root may run more horizontally (e.g. if there is disc degeneration or osteoarthritic change of the exit foramina). In such cases, the safe triangle may not exist and it is safer to deposit the injectate rostral to the nerve root. Pre-procedure MRI studies should be available to assist. Thus there are two procedures for depositing either LA alone (diagnostic block) or LA and steroid (therapeutic block); these are termed the subpedicular and rostral (infraneural) techniques.

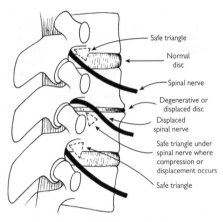

Fig. 4.3 Safe triangle below the pedicle. Note that this triangle can change in degenerative conditions.

Techniques

Subpedicular

With the patient prone obtain a fluoroscopic AP view with cephalocaudal tilt to square off the vertebral endplate closest to the target point (Fig. 4.4). The midpoint of the lower border of the pedicle is the needle entry site. If the lamina obscures entry to the intervertebral foramen, increase the obliquity of the C-arm until it moves medially out of the way. If the superior articular process (SAP) of the pedicle is obscuring entry, further cephalocaudal tilt and/or oblique rotation of the X-ray beam may be needed. Needle entry is from below the pedicle using a down-the-needle ('bull's eye') view. For the less experienced operator it is safer to aim to hit the lower end of the pedicle and then navigate the needle inferiorly below the pedicle just lateral to the 6 o'clock position of the pedicle into the safe triangle. This can be better facilitated with a curved tipped needle. A lateral X-ray view is obtained before advancing the needle into the upper third of the intervertebral foramen. Check a straight AP view; the needle should lie under the pedicle and just lateral to the 6 o'clock position of the pedicle (Fig. 4.5).

Attach a low-volume tube to the needle and inject non-ionic contrast in true AP view to demonstrate the dye spread along the nerve root and the epidural spread and rule out inadvertent vascular injection (Fig. 4.6). Rapid medial spread of the contrast indicates intravascular spread and demands abandonment of the procedure. If the contrast passes laterally, the needle should be adjusted to lie more medially. Inject a small volume of LA for diagnostic purposes; the volume is guided by the amount of contrast needed to outline the nerve root, typically 0.3–0.5mL. If this is a therapeutic injection, combine LA with a steroid. At the lumbar level there is currently a debate about the use of particulate and non-particulate steroids, but at the cervical level it is recommended that only non-particulate steroids such as dexamethasone are used.

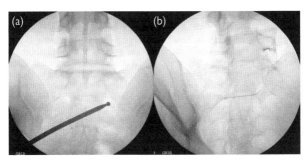

Fig. 4.4 (a) AP view showing squared L5S1 endplates. The S1 foramen can easily be identified. (b) Oblique view showing the needle entry point for S1 and L5 dorsal root block.

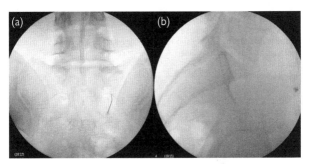

Fig. 4.5 (a) AP view of the needle in the S1 foramen. (b) Lateral view showing the needle tip at the target points in both the S1 and L5 dorsal roots.

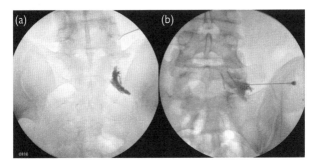

Fig. 4.6 AP views showing good contrast spread to (a) the S1 nerve root and (b) the L5 nerve root.

Rostral (infraneural approach)

Obtain a fluoroscopic AP view with cephalocaudal obliquity to square off the vertebral endplate closest to the target point. Rotate the C-arm obliquely to the side where the procedure is to be performed. Observe the SAP of the vertebra below and align it at about the 6 o'clock position of the inferior border of the pedicle above. The needle entry point is over the SAP of the vertebra below (Fig. 4.7(a)). Use a curved tipped needle as this helps to navigate the needle better. After hitting the SAP in oblique view, navigate the needle tip laterally off the SAP. Then advance the needle in the lateral view to enter the intervertebral foramen. The needle tip is likely to lie in the infraneural position (Fig. 4.7(b)). If the patient complains of radicular pain during advancement of the needle, it may be going more laterally and may have to be advanced more medially hugging the SAP, which is facilitated by using a curved tip needle.

Attach a low-volume tube to the needle and inject non-ionic contrast in true AP view to demonstrate the nerve root and epidural spread. Rapid medial spread of the contrast indicates intravascular spread and demands abandonment of the procedure. If the contrast passes laterally, the needle should be adjusted to lie more medially. Inject a small volume of LA for diagnostic purposes; the volume is guided by the amount of contrast needed to outline the nerve root, typically 0.3–0.5mL. If this is a therapeutic injection, combine LA with a steroid.

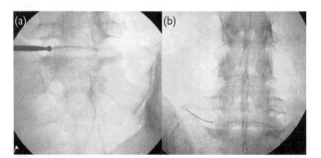

Fig. 4.7 (a) Oblique view—the target point is just above the SAP. (b) AP view showing the needle in position (infraneural approach) for L5 dorsal nerve root block.

Complications and management

Specific complications of this procedure include prolonged nerve conduction block, nerve injury, infection, intravascular injection, and intrathecal injection. Prolonged nerve conduction block may manifest as sensory loss with or without motor weakness for a few hours in the affected dermatome/myotome that outlasts the recovery period. This may impair the patient's ability to function safely. It can be minimized by observing the flow of contrast and volume required to cover the dorsal root and using a similar volume of LA. Some patients appear to be more sensitive to this complication, and it is advisable to warn patients of this possibility. In rare instances it lasts more than 24h. Observation is needed until the patient is safe to mobilize. Nerve injury is rare although paraesthesia during needle placement is fairly common. It is likely that this complication can be minimized by attention to procedural details to avoid inadvertent paraesthesia. Experienced operators recognize radiological landmarks, require fewer needle redirections, and gain feedback. Thus needle entry should have fewer complications. If paraesthesiae occur it is important to withdraw the needle. It is essential to observe for pain during injection since intraneural injection increases the risk of nerve injury and prolonged symptoms.

There have been reports of permanent neurological injury following these procedures, and this has been hypothesized to be associated with particulate depot steroids. This may be due to injection into radicular arteries and subsequent occlusion of end arterial supply of the spinal cord. Although there is evidence to support therapeutic efficacy for non-particulate steroids, the degree of such support is less than with the particulate steroids. Nevertheless, it is advisable to avoid particulate steroids in the light of these possible risks.

Infection is a risk with any invasive procedure and sterile technique is important to minimize this. It is not generally necessary to use prophylactic antibiotics, but an environment with sufficient air changes, antiseptic skin cleansing agent, sterile drapes, sterile needles, and drugs is required. Expertise in the procedure which minimizes the number of needle entries and the time required should lessen the risk of infection. Intra-vascular entry can occur and needle aspiration is recommended before injection. However, aspiration is not always positive despite a needle's being intravascular. Contrast injection may show this by digital subtraction methods. However, if digital subtraction is not available, injecting the contrast in AP view under continuous fluoroscopy and observing the contrast spread may identify vascular spread if the contrast rapidly disappears medially. This can occur in any patient, but may be more common after spinal surgery.

Epidural injection can lead to a more widespread temporary sensory and motor block affecting mobility. Spinal injection can have similar effects but of a more profound nature. It may be associated with vascular collapse from sympathetic blockade which requires resuscitation. This will also depend on the volume and concentration of LA used.

Lumbar facet blocks

Low back pain (LBP) is the most common musculoskeletal disorder of industrialized society and the most common cause of disability in persons younger than 45 years. The facet joints are reported to be the cause of pain in 15–40% cases of LBP. The facet joints are a pair of joints in the posterior aspect of the spine; they are more properly termed the zygapophyseal joints (abbreviated as Z-joints), a term derived from the Greek roots zygos, meaning yoke or bridge, and physis, meaning outgrowth.

Diagnosis of facet joint pain

LBP originating from the facet joints can be difficult to differentiate from other causes of back pain as there are no specific features in the history, examination, or imaging that can reliably predict facet joint pain. The diagnosis can only be confirmed with precision diagnostic blocks.

Although no single sign or symptom is diagnostic, it has been demonstrated that the combination of the following seven factors was significantly correlated with pain relief from an intra-articular facet joint injection:

- older age
- previous history of LBP
- normal gait
- maximal pain with extension from a fully flexed position
- absence of leg pain, but pain may be referred to hip or thigh
- absence of muscle spasm
- absence of exacerbation with a Valsalva manoeuvre.

Examination

Assessment

- Posture: there may be loss of lumbar lordosis.
- Muscles: evidence of muscle spasm or wasting, use of muscle groups to maintain posture.
- Joints: range of movement, pain on movement, tender points. With facet-joint-mediated LBP, pain is often increased with hyperextension or rotation of the lumbar spine, and it might be either focal or radiating. There may be an abnormal pelvic tilt and rotation of the hip secondary to tight hamstrings, hip rotators, and quadrates, but these findings are non-specific.
- Nerves: check for lower-limb neurological deficit. Sensations are usually normal in these patients, as are motor power and reflexes.

Investigation

- X-rays: may show degenerative changes but are not diagnostic.
- CT scan: may show facet joint pathology even in asymptomatic patients and so is not useful in diagnosis.
- MRI: useful to exclude disc pathology and neural compromise.

Medial branch blocks

Fluoroscopically guided medial branch nerve injections are used for diagnostic purposes to determine whether the facet joint in question is responsible for the LBP. Injections are diagnostic if patients report significant relief of symptoms (usually at least a 50% reduction in pain).

Anatomy

Facet joints are formed by the articulation of the SAPs of one vertebra with the inferior articular processes of the vertebra above. The two common mechanisms for pain generation in the lumbar facet joints are either direct, from an arthritic process within the joint itself, or indirect, where overgrowth of the joint (e.g. hypertrophy or a synovial cyst) impinges on nearby structures.

The dorsal ramus divides into three branches termed medial, lateral, and intermediate. The medial branch innnervates the facet joints, giving off two branches to the nearby facet joints. One branch innervates the facet joint at that level, and the second branch descends caudally to the level below. Therefore each medial branch of the dorsal ramus innervates two joints—that level and the level below (e.g. the L3 medial branch innervates the L3/4 and L4/5 facet joints). Similarly, each facet joint is innervated by the two most cephalad medial branches (e.g. the L3/L4 facet joint is innervated by the L2/L3 medial branch. (See Fig. 1.1.)

Contraindications

Absolute
- Bacterial infection (systemic or localized in the region of the block)
- Bleeding diathesis
- Possible pregnancy.

Relative
- Allergy to contrast media(may be done with steroid cover)
- Allergy to LA (sometimes can use alternative LA)
- Concurrent treatment with aspirin or NSAIDS that may compromise coagulation
- Neurological disorders (other than radicular pain).

Patient position

Diagnostic blocks can be performed using a posterior or an oblique approach to the lumbar spine. The oblique approach is the most convenient and the least technically demanding. The patient can be positioned as follows.
- Prone with oblique view obtained by rotating the C-arm of the fluoroscope
- Semi-prone with a pillow under the abdomen to tilt the target side upwards.

Target identification

The target point for the the L1–L4 medial branches will be at the junction of the SAP and the transverse process which the target nerve crosses midway between the superior border of the transverse process and the location of the mamillo-accessory notch.

At the L5 level, the target nerve is not the medial branch but the L5 dorsal ramus.

In the oblique view the target point lies above and behind the 'eye' of the 'scotty dog' or the midpoint of the line between the ventral edge of the SAP and the mamillo-accessory notch.

L1–L4 medial branch blocks

In the oblique view, a puncture point is selected by placing the tip of the needle in a tunnel view to the X-ray beam, with the target point behind the 'eye' of the 'scotty dog'.

The progress of the needle is monitored by intermittent screening and stopped when its tip strikes the bone. This should be at the neck of SAP. Correct placement is confirmed in AP view where the tip of the needle should be at least opposite to the lateral margin of the silhouette of the SAP and preferably slightly medial to the margin. Once in the correct position, the needle bevel should be directed caudally to avoid spread of the drug into the intervertebral foramen.

Dose

0.1–0.3mL of contrast is injected to confirm position and lack of venous uptake, and then 0.5mL is injected onto the target nerve. Both nerves innervating the joint are injected.

L5 dorsal ramus blocks

Target identification

The same protocol as previously described is used except that the target nerve is not the medial branch but the dorsal ramus itself. The target point is the junction of the ala of the sacrum with the SAP of the sacrum.

The target point is seen in AP views as a notch between these two bones (Fig. 4.8b).

Needle placement

The puncture point in the skin is just lateral to the target point, so the course of the needle is anterior and medial and should remain medial to the adjacent iliac crest. The progress of the needle is monitored by intermittent screening and stopped when the tip strikes the bone. Correct placement is confirmed in the AP view as the needle is tucked against the SAP of the sacrum and under its lateral margin. Once the needle is in position, the bevel is directed to face medially to reduce the risk of inadvertent spread of drug into the L5–S1 intervertebral or S1 posterior forama.

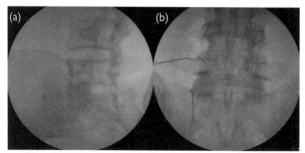

Fig. 4.8 (a) Oblique view showing the needle at the L4 medial branch. (b) AP view showing the needle in position at the L5 dorsal ramus in the sacral notch. The L4 medial block needle can also be seen on the AP view at the junction between the SAP and the mamillo-accessory notch.

Lumbar facet joint injection

Intra-articular facet blocks can be considered for facetogenic pain, but according to the current ISIS guidelines lumbar medial branch blocks should replace intra-artcular injections as they are safer to perform, more expedient, more easily subject to control, and of more therapeutic utility in that, if positive, the pain can be treated with RF neurotomy.

Complications

- Vasovagal syncope
- Bleeding
- Infection
- Post-procedural radicular pain
- Dural puncture and post dural puncture headache
- Allergic reaction to medication

In reality the risk of damage to other structures is unlikely if small movements are made under fluoroscopic control with perfect alignment of the image.

Intravascular injection is unlikely if the needle tip is placed accurately. Misdirection of the needle can result in placing the needle intradurally or onto the nerve root if the image is not perfectly aligned.

Assessment

Record the patient's self-assessment of pain, mobility, and radiation pattern before and after the diagnostic block. Assessments can be made immediately after the block and on the following days. Benefit may extend beyond the expected duration of effect of the LA used.

Further reading

Bogduk N (2004). *Practice Guidelines for Spinal Diagnostic and Treatment Procedures.* San Francisco, CA: ISIS.

Jackson RP, Jacobs RR, Montesano PX (1988) Volvo award in clinical sciences. Facet joint injection in low-back pain. A prospective statistical study. Spine. Sep 1988;13(9):966–71.

Lumbosacral facet syndrome. http://emedicine.medscape.com/article/94871-overview.

Rathmell J (2006). *Atlas of Image-Guided Interventions.* Baltimore, MD: Lippincott–Williams & Wilkins.

Waldman S (2009). *Atlas of Interventional Pain Management* (3rd edn). Philadelphia, PA: WB Saunders.

Lumbar facet radiofrequency denervation

Indications

Radiofrequency (RF) denervation may help back pain with or with out radiation that can be eliminated by a local anaesthetic block of the medial branch of the dorsal ramus at the levels of pain.

Patient selection

Patients who have had constant back ache for at least 6 months where conservative measures have not helped. Back pain usually arises in middle age or later, often after exertion or asymmetrical strain, but can occur in the teens and twenties as a result of trauma. Pain is often worse while standing still, sitting in or getting up from a soft sofa, and long walks. Patients usually complain of having more pain in the mornings, which becomes better as they 'get going'. It is common for patients to complain of a patchy diffuse radiation (non-dermatomal) down the leg that may go all the way to the foot and is often mistakenly interpreted as radicular. Previous surgery or RF neurotomy are not a contraindication. These patients have less pain if they keep moving about and take short walks.

Clinical examination

If the patient is examined with light coming from the side or directly above, prominence of the paravertebral muscles may become apparent. Mark the upper limit of the tense swollen muscles as all these levels will need to be tested. Paravertebral tenderness is usually accentuated by spinal extension; this test (facet compression) often provokes radiation of pain down the leg. There is often reduced sensation along the outside of the leg. It is common to find weakness or absence of ankle reflex on the painful side.

Investigations

The diagnosis can be confirmed by performing medial branch blocks using small volumes (1mL) of LA injection(s) to the medial branch of the dorsal ramus, taking care to avoid intravascular injections as this will give a false-negative conclusion. To reduce the risk of entering a blood vessel either withdraw the needle a few millimetres whilst injecting or test with contrast before injecting the LA. Careful assessment of pain after the blocks is essential; a positive result is suggested by 80–100% relief following injection, lasting at least for the duration expected from the LA used. In practice, there is great variation and it is common to have complete pain relief for a day or two with both bupivacaine and lidocaine. To reduce the risk of a placebo response, two clearly positive blocks on two separate occasions are considered sufficient to establish the diagnosis. As each joint is supplied by two nerves, one at the same level and one from above, it is necessary to inject both levels. It is recommended that a minimum of three nerves (two joints) are injected, and possibly more depending on how high up the back muscle spasm was observed prior to injection.

Contraindications

Absolute
- Patient unwilling
- Infection at the site of treatment
- Pregnancy, bleeding disorders, and anticoagulants
- Previous surgery or RF neurotomies *are not* a contraindication

Relative
- Patients with significant psychological problems may be unsuitable.
- Cardiac pacemakers—it is important to keep the cardiologist involved and the patients may need cardiac monitoring during the RF denervation.
- Insufficient experience when faced with patients who have advanced degenerative changes where interpretation of the anatomy may be very difficult.

Consent

The patient should be aware that, despite the positive diagnostic blocks, there is no guarantee of pain relief following the procedure. They must be aware that cooperation during the procedure is imperative and that communication between doctor and patient is maintained. The procedure will require the patient to be aware so that they can report any unexpected symptom immediately. They must be told that there could be pain from the procedure, that the immediate postoperative period requires care, and that they need to avoid heavy work.

Preparation

The procedure is peformed in a room that is suitable for an aseptic procedure with fluoroscopy C-arm facilities and a narrow radio-translucent table (ideally 50cm) which allows free movement of the C-arm so that the X-ray beam can be directed from all angles. Operators must be familiar with the RF generator. They must be trained in the use of fluoroscopy to obtain the best images and thereby have reliable information about electrode positions. Lidocaine is used to anaesthetize skin and muscles and bupivacaine 0.5% for the target nerve prior to lesioning.

Position

The patient lies prone on the X-ray table with pillows appropriately placed for comfort. Sometimes putting a pillow under the hip on the side to be treated, especially when treating the left side, can be advantageous as this moves the tube of the C-arm away from the operator's head. The operator stands on the patient's left, the C-arm should be on the patient's right, and the X-ray monitor is close to the patient's head but still on the other side of the table from the operator. If the operator is left-handed, everything can be reversed.

Technique

Knowledge of the anatomy of the dorsal rami and medial branches that supply the facet joints is essential before embarking on this procedure. The most important anatomical feature(s) is the slope of the superior and posterior aspect(s) of the medial part of the transverse process at the

L1–L5 levels. The target nerve (medial branch of the dorsal ramus) lies along this slope, hugging the base of the SAP and travelling posteriorly and downwards towards the lower end of the facet joint. The dorsal ramus devides into the lateral, intermediate, and medial branches at the anterior edge of the articular process. The medial branch that is the target nerve disappears under the mamillo-accessory ligament at the posterior part of the side of the base of the articular process. The area where it is accessible is in the middle of the side of the articular process. At the lowest level, the dorsal ramus of L5 lies over the ala of the sacrum, hugging the base of the SAP arising from the sacrum and forming the L5/S1 joint with the inferior articular process of L5. The dorsal ramus does not divide into the medial and lateral branches until after it has reached the lower end of the joint. Thus at the L5/S1 level the dorsal ramus rather than the medial branch is the target nerve. The aim is to have the cannula lying parallel to these nerves and to make two or three closely spaced lesions in the area to 'carpet' the nerve. An 18G cannula with a bent 10mm non-insulated tip is recommended; two adjacent lesions will usually suffice. A finer cannula can be used, but the lesions are smaller and therefore more lesions will be required, adding to the time taken.

A number of steps are required to perform the RF procedure and to position the cannula in the shortest possible time with absolute certainty. To get the needle parallel to the nerve it is necessary to come from below at about 15°–20° lateral to the saggital plane. In practice this is achieved by getting the best view from the most caudal angle of the curvature that is formed by the upper border of the transverse process as it comes medially and then goes up along the lateral border of the SAP. The point where the cannula punctures the skin is crucial in achieving a satisfactory position for lesioning. If followed meticulously, the following steps will make RF relatively easy. Adjust the C-arm to obtain a perfect AP view of the lower lumbar spine, including the upper border of the sacrum. Swing the C-arm in a cephalad direction, maintaining the AP view, to see the L5/S1 disc (this may be much further than you think). This view will enable identification of the L5 vertebrae with absolute certainty.

The methods for performing lesions at the base of the articular processes from L5 and upwards are all identical.

Bring the C-arm back, slightly to eliminate the double shadow of the upper endplate of the L5 vertebral body (i.e. 'square up'). The transverse process of L5 should now be halfway between the upper and lower endplates. Rotate the C-arm laterally to see the facet joint space; this provides a good view of the curvature. Bring the C-arm downwards (caudal) and medially (until it is 15°–20° lateral to the sagittal plane) while maintaining a good view of the curvature. If the SAP is hyper-trophic, the curvature will be lost sooner than expected whilst bringing the C-arm medially. If this occurs, move laterally again until the curvature comes back into view. The cannula insertion will take a direction that is more lateral (25°–35° from the sagittal plane), aiming medially towards the groove where the nerve lies. It is essential to realize that if the cannula comes from a more medial angle, either it will get stuck on the hypertrophied process or it will be deflected laterally and miss the nerve altogether (Fig. 4.9). Once the best view of the curvature has obtained (looking from below), make a mark on the skin with a felt pen a little below the medial part of the curve (Fig. 4.10(a)).

After skin anaesthesia is achieved, insert the cannula using the 'tunnel' technique (needle in the direction of the X-ray beam so that it appears as a dot); it is vital to make bone contact (Fig. 4.10(b)). Inject small amounts of LA as required. After bone contact is made, the cannula can be gently manoeuvred up to the upper edge of the transverse process but no further.

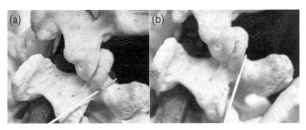

Fig. 4.9 (a) and (b) show what happens when approaching the medial branch from an angle that does not compensate for the hypertrophic superior articular process: (a) the cannula is deflected laterally and will not lie along the nerve; (b) the cannula is placed from a slightly more lateral angle which then allows it to lie along the nerve at the base of the articular process.

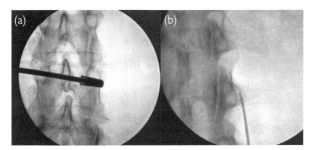

Fig. 4.10 (a) Skin insertion point for L3 medial branch (on L4 transverse process). (b) Bone contact on L4 transverse process.

There are three fluoroscopy views which can confirm the correct and safe position of the cannula. If it is inserted too far, beyond the upper edge of the transverse process, it will reach the anterior ramus (ventral root). This must never happen.

- Inferior 'tunnel' view: having placed the cannula as described, bring the C-arm slightly caudal (downwards) to see the cannula from below in close contact with the bone in the curvature (Fig. 4.11(a)).

- Oblique view: bring the C-arm back to the AP position and then rotate it laterally, keeping the cannula at about 8 o'clock on the monitor, and again check that the tip is just short of the anterior edge of the articular process (Fig. 4.11(b)).
- Superior view: move the C-arm in a cephalad direction as far as it will go, maintaining the cannula in a 6 o'clock position, to be able to see the superior surface of the transverse process. The tip of the cannula must not extend all the way up to the upper edge of the transverse process; it is essential to maintain some space between the tip of the cannula and the upper edge in this view (Fig. 4.11(c)).

Remove the stylet from the cannula and insert the electrode. Check that the cannula has not moved during this process. Make sure that the earth plate is in firm contact with the skin and that the RF generator indicates that connections are intact. Stimulation is not necessary to confirm the correct position as this has been done using the different X-ray views described. Perform the first lesion. Use the automatic mode on the RF generator, and set the temperature at 85°C and the duration to 65–70s. This allows time to reach the set temperature and then produce a 60s lesion. After this lesion the electrode can be shifted a couple of millimetres either medially or laterally depending on where on the curve the first lesion was made. Carefully check the electrode position again using all three views before making a second lesion. Two lesions using an 18G cannula with a 10mm tip are usually sufficient; a third lesion can be made if it is felt that coverage of the target area was not achieved with two lesions.

The lesions at the base of the articular processes from L5 and upwards are all identical. Medial branches of the dorsal rami of L4 and upwards will have been lesioned.

The lesion at the ala of the sacrum on the side of the base of the articular process that forms the L5/S1 joint will target the L5 dorsal ramus. This is very important as the lowest two facet joints that are most often (but not always) the cause of symptoms especially in middle and old age.

The technique is basically the same. Start by visualizing the L5 vertebral body and remove the double shadow of the lower endplate as much as possible. Rotate the C-arm laterally to see the joint space of the L5/S1 joint; this may need to be quite far laterally. The iliac crest will move medially as the C-arm rotates and cover the target. Familiarity with the individual anatomy of the patient (there is great variation) may give, with experience, an approximate indication of the best skin puncture point. Return the C-arm medially; the iliac crest will move laterally and expose the curvature. It looks like a valley formed by the lateral edge of the articular process coming down to the upper surface of the ala of the sacrum and then ascending laterally. Move the C-arm in a caudal (downwards) direction while maintaining a good view of the 'valley' until it starts to become less clear. Return the C-arm upwards until the good view of the curvature is restored. The puncture point is then marked just below the valley (Fig. 4.12(a)).

The cannula is introduced after skin anaesthesia using the 'tunnel' technique until bone contact is made. The cannula is then advanced to the edge of the valley and the same three views are used to confirm correct and safe placement (Fig. 4.12(b)–(d)). Two adjacent lesions should be made.

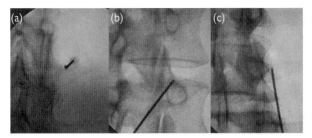

Fig. 4.11 (a) Inferior tunnel view to confirm cannula tip in contact with bone. (b) Posterolateral view with cannula at 8 o'clock to confirm tip just short of upper edge of transverse process, 4 o'clock when doing left side. (c) Cephalad view with cannula at 6 o'clock looking from above to confirm tip just short of anterior border of transverse process.

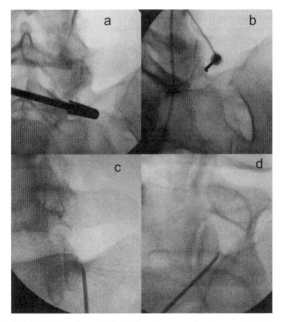

Fig. 4.12 (a) Skin insertion point for L5 dorsal ramus on ala of sacrum. (b) Inferior tunnel view to confirm cannula tip in contact with bone. (c) Cephalad view with cannula at 6 o'clock looking from above to confirm tip just short of anterior border. (d) Posterolateral view with cannula at 8 o'clock to confirm that the cannula is not inserted beyond the anterior edge of the articular process.

Post-procedure management

It is common to have increased pain which may last from a few days to a few weeks after RF denervation. It is very important that the patient is aware of this and is given analgesia and support. The patient needs to avoid heavy exertion after RF, and if daily work involves a significant amount of lifting or physical exertion then a week or two off work may be justified. Follow-up at regular intervals (usually 1, 3, 6, and 12 months) is advised and can be done by telephone. Some or all of the pain may recur after some months or years. It is quite easy to confirm the cause of the pain and treat with RF again, and is usually successful.

Complications

Complications are extremely rare if the procedure is performed correctly and with attention to detail. Infection, bleeding, and allergic reaction to LA are theoretically possible but have not been reported. The main risk is inserting the electrode too far onto the ventral ramus. However, even this will not cause damage if the patient is awake and immediately reports burning down the leg and the operator aborts the lesion. Some radiation of pain down the leg during lesioning is common, but as long as the electrode position has been confirmed to be correct there is no problem. Retracting the electrode a few millimetres until the pain stops will only result in failure to coagulate the medial branch and give an unsatisfactory result.

Pearls of wisdom

- Probably the most common cause of failure is treatment of an insufficient number of levels. It is better to treat an extra level, and sometimes even extend to the upper lumbar area, than to try and limit the number of levels to the minimum.
- There is an intimate relationship between the dorsal ramus, the ventral ramus, and the sympathetic chain. When the results of RF are unsatisfactory and further medial branch blocks do not eliminate residual pain, sympathetically mediated pain and a radicular component should be considered. Diagnostic sympathetic and/or selective root block (trans-foraminal injection) may assist with diagnosis. It is important to remember that radicular pain components do not always involve the whole dermatome; the patient may complain of pain only in the thigh, buttock, or calf.

Sacroiliac joint interventions

Anatomy

The sacroiliac joint (SIJ) is the largest axial joint in the body, with an average surface area of $17.5cm^2$. It is a true synovial joint with a fibrous capsule. The joint is also supported by a network of muscles that help to deliver regional muscular forces to the pelvic bones. Some of these muscles, such as the gluteus maximus, piriformis, and biceps femoris, are functionally connected to SIJ ligaments, so their actions can affect joint mobility.

The joint is flat until puberty, after which coarse ridges and depressions develop by the age of 30 years with accelerated changes after the age of 50 years. The synovial cleft narrows to 1–2mm iat age 50–70 years and to 0–1mm at age >70 years. However, complete intra-articular ankylosis is relatively rare.

A cadaver study showed that the joint is innervated posteriorly from the lateral branches of the S1–S4 dorsal rami. Other studies have shown predominant dorsal innervation of the joint in humans with sensory fibres from the L5 dorsal ramus and the S1–S4 dorsal rami. An anatomical study of cadavers demonstrated that the number and location of lateral branches from each sacral dorsal ramus to the SIJ complex displayed marked variation. The lateral branches exited from the 2 o'clock to the 6 o'clock positions on the right, and from the 6 o'clock to the 10 o'clock positions on the left at the S1–S3 foramen dorsally. This study also reported that on lateral branch differential sensory stimulation in patients with SIJ pain diagnosed by SIJ injection all patients demonstrated identifiable symptomatic branches stemming from both the L5 dorsal ramus and the S1 dorsal ramus, 78% had a symptomatic lateral branch from S2, and 42% had a symptomatic lateral branch from S3. The prevalence of SIJ pain in carefully screened LBP patients appears to range from 15% to 25%.

Causes of SIJ pain are intra-articular (e.g. arthritis, infection) and extra-articular (e.g. enthesopathy, fractures, ligamentous injury, myofascial pain). Clinical studies have demonstrated significant pain relief after both intra-articular and peri-articular SIJ injections.

Risk factors that increase the stress borne by the SIJ include true and apparent leg-length discrepancy, gait abnormalities, prolonged vigorous exercise, scoliosis, and spinal fusion to the sacrum. Pregnancy predisposes women to SIJ pain via the combination of increased weight gain, exaggerated lordotic posture, the mechanical trauma of parturition, and hormone-induced ligament laxity. Inflammation of one or both SIJs is an early and prominent symptom in all seronegative and HLA-B27-associated spondylarthropathies.

Diagnosis and treatment

Of all signs of SIJ pain, maximum pain below L5 coupled with pointing to the posterior superior iliac spine (PSIS) or tenderness just medial to the PSIS (sacral sulcus tenderness) have the highest positive predictive value (60%). If these signs are absent, the likelihood of SIJ pain is <10%.

Conservative treatment includes managing psychological issues and addressing leg-length discrepancy with sole raises or pharmacotherapy for connective tissue causes. If the pain does not settle with conservative management, intra-articular injection with local anaesthesia and steroid often serves the dual function of aiding diagnosis and being therapeutic. Most, but not all, investigators have found that radiologically guided SIJ injections provide good pain relief. There are many studies demonstrating prolonged pain relief after intra-articular SIJ steroid injections. Double-blind studies have also shown a beneficial effect for peri-articular cortico-steroid treatment.

SIJ injections are not accurate when performed without guidance. In a double-blind study in 37 patients (39 joints) to determine the accuracy of clinically guided SIJ injections using CT imaging as the standard, it was found that intra-articular injection was accomplished in only 22% of patients, whereas sacral foraminal spread occurred in 44%. In three patients, no contrast was seen on CT scanning, indicating probable vascular uptake. In 24% of injections, contrast extended into the epidural space.

Fluoroscopic-guided injection of local anaesthetic into the SIJ or over the nerve supply of the SIJ can assist diagnosis. However, most clinicians tend to use a mixture of LA and a steroid; this aids diagnosis and in some patients provides good pain relief for weeks and sometimes months although the primary aim of the procedure is diagnostic.

SIJ injection technique

Fluoroscopic guidance is required and the beam is tilted cephalo-caudal so that it is perpendicular to the sacrum. Two techniques have been described.

- The C-arm is angled obliquely (generally 50–100° to the contralateral side) so that the posterior and anterior SIJ lines are overlapped to obtain a radiolucent line along the joint. A curved tipped spinal needle is then inserted into the lower end of the SIJ. Contrast is injected to confirm correct placement of the needle (Figs. 4.13 and 4.14).
- In the other technique the anterior and the posterior SIJ lines are separated. The medial joint lines normally correspond to the posterior joint lines in the AP view. The posterior joint lines are aligned with continuous fluoroscopy to obtain a zone of maximum radiolucency. The inferior part of the joint line is entered with a curved tipped spinal needle.

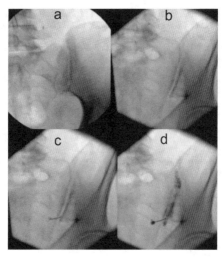

Fig. 4.13 (a, b) AP SIJ: the medial joint line is the posterior joint line. The anterior and posterior joint lines have been aligned using contralateral oblique rotation. (c, d) A 22G needle with a curved tip is seen entering the inferior part of the SIJ and contrast injection confirms the correct needle tip position (Reproduced from Gupta S, Richardson J (2009). *Sacroiliac Joint Block*. In: *Interventional Pain Management: A Practical Approach*, eds. Baneti, Bakshi, Gupta, Gehdoo, Figures 27.1 to 27.4, with permission from Jaypee Brothers Medical Publishers.)

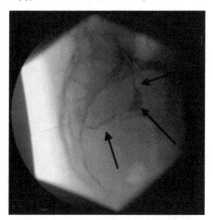

Fig. 4.14 Contrast spread can be seen along the perimeter of the joint line in lateral view as marked by arrows. (Reproduced from Gupta S, Richardson J (2009). *Sacroiliac Joint Block*. In: *Interventional Pain Management: A Practical Approach*, eds. Baneti, Bakshi, Gupta, Gehdoo, Figure 27.5, with permission from Jaypee Brothers Medical Publishers.)

Injection of contrast is mandatory to confirm correct needle tip placement before injection into the SIJ. However, if the needle tip is not in the SIJ after injecting contrast, further needle placement can be difficult if not impossible. To address this problem a double-needle technique has been described for SIJ injections in difficult cases. Once the tip of the needle is correctly placed, its position is checked under continuous fluoroscopy while moving the C-arm in the right and left oblique directions. With continuous fluoroscopy, the tip of the needle should remain within the joint lines and not appear to be on the bone. If the tip of the needle moves away from the joint line, a new SIJ line should be identified by continuous fluoroscopy and another needle advanced into the newly identified joint line (Fig. 4.15(a, b)). Continuous fluoroscopy is repeated to confirm that the tip of the second needle remains within the joint lines. Once both needles are in place, contrast is injected through the needle that is most likely to be in the joint (Fig. 4.15(c, d)). If contrast spread is not satisfactory, contrast is injected through the other needle.

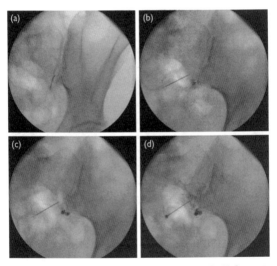

Fig. 4.15 (a) A curved tipped needle is advanced into the right SIJ. (b) On continuous fluoroscopy the tip of the needle appears to be on the bone. With continuous fluoroscopy another translucent joint area is identified and a second needle is advanced into the joint. (c) Contrast is injected through the second needle and the SIJ is outlined. (d) Contrast injected through the first needle shows contrast spreading medially—possibly a vascular spread. (Reprinted with permission from *Pain Physician* journal and the American Society of Interventional Pain Physicians. S Gupta. 'Double Needle Technique: An Alternative Method for Performing Difficult SIJ Injections.' *Pain Physician* 2011; **14**: 281–4.

Radiofrequency denervation of SIJ

Several investigators have performed RF denervation procedures to provide prolonged pain relief to patients with SIJ pain. The techniques used have ranged from denervating nerves supplying the SIJ to creating lesions in the joint itself. The success in studies targeting the nerve supply is higher than in those focusing on the joint. The major drawback to percutaneous RF denervation procedures is that they should not be expected to alleviate pain emanating from the ventral SIJ. A further complication is that the nerves lesioned during RF procedures innervate other pain-generating structures as well as the SIJ, and the SIJ is probably innervated by other nerves which are inaccessible for denervation.

Techniques for RF denervation of SIJ

Several techniques for RF neurotomy of the SIJ have been advocated.

Sensory-stimulation-guided lateral branch RF neurotomy

This has been carried out using standard RF needles and technique and stimulating the lateral branch nerves at S1, S2, and S3 (Fig. 4.16) and also the L5 posterior sensory branches. Studies show that 64–88% patients had >50% pain relief at 6–9-month follow-up and 36% were pain free at 6 months follow-up.

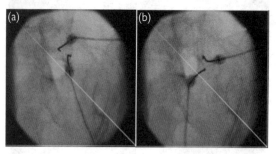

Fig. 4.16 Needle placement for sensory-stimulation-guided lateral branch RF neurotomy.

Bipolar lateral branch RF

Two electrodes are placed lateral to the sacral foramina of S1, S2, and S3. An inter-electrode distance of 4–6mm for bipolar lesions has been shown to be the maximum effective distance for creating a continuous strip lesion. A prospective cohort study has been performed.

Pulsed RF

This has been attempted in one prospective study (22 patients). Pulsed RF (perpendicular approach) was performed at the L4 medial branch and L5 dorsal root, and sensory stimulation was used for lateral branch localization at S1 and S2. Two pulsed lesions (second rotated 180°) were performed at 45V for 120s at 39–42°C. Almost three-quarters had a drop of >50% in Visual Analogue Scale (VAS) with a mean duration of relief of 20 weeks.

SInergy™ cooled RF technique
This allows much larger lesions to be generated than seen with standard RF. The volume of a cooled RF lesion is equivalent to that of 8–10 standard RF lesions. There is clearly an advantage to having larger predictable lesions to ablate the lateral branch nerves at S1, S2, and S3 because their anatomical positions may vary and are unpredictably located by traditional sensory testing. Since the cooled RF lesion is also concentric it is more reliable at projecting a lesion on the uneven surface of the sacrum. The active tip is cooled to 60°C using a water pump. This allows predictable expansion of the lesion over a 2.5min cycle. Nine lesions are created: one at the L5 medial branch, three each at S1 and S2, and two at S3. Lesions should be 8–10mm from the lateral edge of the foramina (Fig. 4.17).

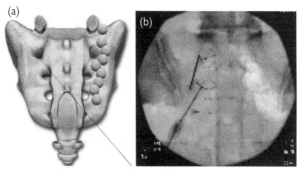

Fig. 4.17 Site of lesions for SInergy™ cooled RF technique.

Simplicity™ technique
A curved RF probe is placed along the posterior plate of the sacrum lateral to the S1–S3 foramen as shown in Fig. 4.18 and the lesion is performed. The L5 dorsal rami are denervated using the conventional technique (Fig. 4.18). If the RF generator does not have the Simplicity™ or cooled RF facility, an 18G needle can be used and the tip insulation is stripped to 1 inch active tip. This can then be placed in the line netween the sacral foramen and the SI joint as shown in Fig. 4.19.

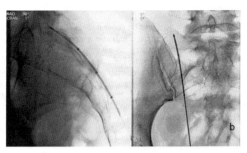

Fig. 4.18 (a) AP view of the Simplicity™ probe in place. (b) Lateral view of the Simplicity™ probe in use.

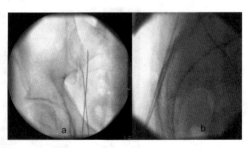

Fig. 4.19 (a) AP and (b) lateral views of an 18G needle with a 1 inch active tip placed in the target. This will be moved up to create more lesions covering the whole space between the sacral foramen and the SIJ line.

Further reading

Bogduk N (2004). Sacroiliac joint blocks. In: Bogduk N (ed) *Practice Guidelines: Spinal Diagnostic and Treatment Procedures*, pp.66–86. San Francisco, CA: ISIS.

Buijs EJ, Kamphuis ET, Groen GJ (2004). Radiofrequency treatment of sacroiliac joint-related pain aimed at the first three sacral dorsal rami: a minimal approach. *Pain Clinic* **16**: 139–46.

Burnham RS, Yutaks Y (2007). An alternate method of radiofrequency neurotomy of the sacroiliac joint: a pilot study of the effect on pain, function and satisfaction. *Reg Anesth Pain Med* **32**: 3–6.

Cohen SP, Abdi S (2003). Lateral branch blocks as a treatment for sacroiliac joint pain: a pilot study. *Reg Anesth Pain Med* **28**: 113–19.

Dreyfuss P, Park K, Bogduk N, *et al.* (2000). Do L5 dorsal ramus and S1–4 lateral branch blocks protect the SIJ from an experimental pain stimulus? A randomized, double-blind controlled trial. Presented at the Annual Meeting of ISIS, San Francisco, CA, 2000.

Gupta S (2011). Double needle technique: an alternative method for performing difficult sacroiliac joint injections. *Pain Physician* **14**: 281–4.

Gupta S, Richardson J (2009). Sacroiliac joint block. In: Baheti DK, Bakshi S, Gupta S, Gehdoo RP (eds) *Interventional Pain Management: A Practical Approach*. New Delhi: Jaypee Brothers Medical Publishers.

Ikeda R (1991). Innervation of the sacroiliac joint: microscopic and histological studies. *J Nippon Med School* **58**: 587–96.

Vallejo R, Benyamin RM, Stanton G, *et al.* (2006). Pulsed radiofrequency denervation for the treatment of sacroiliac joint syndrome. *Pain Med* **7**: 429–34.

Yin W, Willard F, Carreiro J, *et al.* (2003). Sensory stimulation-guided sacroiliac joint radio-frequency neurotomy: technique based on neuroanatomy of the dorsal sacral plexus. *Spine* **28**: 2419–25.

Cervical spine interventions

A. Baker, G. Baranidharan, P. Toomey, and S. Nath

Cervical epidural

Anatomy

- Boundaries:
  - superior—fusion of dura at foramen magnum
  - inferior—sacro coccygeal membrane
  - anterior—posterior longitudinal ligament
  - posterior—laminae and ligamentum flavum
  - lateral—pedicles and foraminae.
- Contents: fat, veins and arteries, lymphatics.
- Depth: 3–4 mm at C7/T1 with the neck flexed.
- Path of needle: skin, subcutaneous tissue, ligamentum nuchae, interspinous ligmanent, ligmentum flavum, epidural space. Note that in many patients, the ligamentum flavum may not meet in the midline and the operator might not obtain a true loss of resistance.

Indications

Chronic pain

- Cervical radiculopathy and spondylosis
- Vertebral disc herniation
- Neuropathic pain (diabetic, post-herpetic)
- Complex regional pain syndrome
- Phantom limb pain
- Refractory shoulder and upper-limb pain syndromes
- Malignancy (primary head/neck/upper limb, metastatic, chemotherapy-related).

Acute pain

- Postoperative analgesia (particularly following sternotomy)
- Acute vascular insufficiency
- Acute herpes zoster.

Diagnostic

- Differential blockade to evaluate head/neck/upper-limb pain.

Contraindications

Absolute

- Patient refusal
- Untreated infection at the injection site
- Possible systemic infection
- Bleeding diathesis/anticoagulants.

Relative

- Known immune suppression
- Known anatomically difficult spine.

Positioning

- Sitting (not safe as the patient can have syncopal attacks).
- Prone (preferred for X-ray guidance, care to position neck correctly).
- Lateral (not commonly used).
- Keep arms by the side to obtain appropriate fluoroscopic images.

Technique

- Interlaminar approach.
- Establish IV access.
- Select 16–22G Tuohy needle with a loss of resistance syringe. A 16G needle offers better resistance for inexperienced hands, but is more of a problem if a dural tap occurs.
- Prone position with neck flexed, forehead cushioned, and arms by sides.
- Identify C7/T1 interspace (vertebra prominens is at C7) (Fig. 5.1). An epidural performed above this level can increase the risk of both dural puncture and spinal cord injury.
- Mark interspace with pointer and confirm with AP fluoroscopy projection.
- Use either loss or resistance to saline or air or a hanging-drop technique.
- Inject non-ionic contrast under continuous fluoroscopy. This will show if the contrast has spread onto the desired nerve root (Fig. 5.2).
- Obtain AP, lateral, and oblique fluoroscopy views to confirm epidural needle placement and the spread. This will also help to exclude intra-vascular, subarachnoid, or subdural injection.
- Inject a combination of LA and steroid (5–7mL).

The transforaminal approach is an alternative but will not be discussed further.

Fluoroscopy

- Prone position gives the best AP picture and sitting provides a good lateral view. In the prone position, having the arms by the sides and being pulled down by assistants can take the shoulders away from the active image and provide a better lateral view.

Complications

- Dural puncture ± total spinal
- Postdural puncture headache
- Subdural puncture
- Intravascular injection
- Haematoma
- Infection (e.g. epidural abscess)
- Neurological trauma (direct spinal cord or nerve root damage).

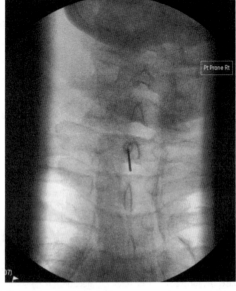

Fig. 5.1 The C7/T1 and T1/2 interspaces.

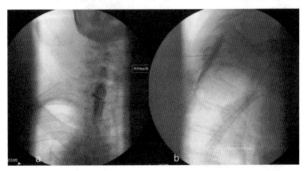

Fig. 5.2 (a) AP and (b) lateral views showing good contrast spread in the epidural space.

Clinical pearls of wisdom

- Always enter at C7/T1 or T1/2. If an MRI scan is available, look at the epidural fat or discuss with the radiologist.
- Positioning is crucial—ensure adequate neck flexion.
- Avoid sedation if possible.
- As cervical ligaments are less substantial than those in the thoracic or lumbar regions, it is common to obtain a false loss of resistance. A lateral view can be helpful.
- Lateral fluoroscopy helps to gauge the depth of the needle tip; it is important not to advance further than the foramina. This can happen, especially if the needle is not in the midline.
- A catheter can be passed through the epidural needle if the target point is higher up in the cervical space. Fill the catheter with contrast to aid navigation.
- Pre-emptive glycopyrrolate 200micrograms can help to prevent vasovagal symptoms that may occur, especially in sitting patients.
- Entering the space with para-median approach and gauging the depth by deliberately hitting the lamina can increase the safety.

Cervical medial branch block

Diagnostic blocks

Cervical spine pain

Cervical spine pain is commonly associated with degenerative processes in the spine or with trauma, most commonly whiplash injury. A number of structures in the neck can contribute to pain symptoms. Pain arising from the facet (zygo-apophyseal) joints can be diagnosed by blocking the median branch of the dorsal ramus supplying the facet joints. Diagnostic blocks should be performed before considering more interventional techniques.

Patient selection

Cervical spine pain originating from the facet joints can be difficult to differentiate from other causes of spinal pain. There are no specific features in the history, examination, or imaging that can reliably predict pain arising from facet joints. The diagnosis can only be confirmed with precision diagnostic blocks.

History

- Axial neck pain.
- Pain affected by posture and movement, particularly neck extension.
- Neck stiffness.
- Referral of pain. There is a non-specific radiation pattern (Fig. 5.3):
  - upper (C2/3) cervical facet pain often referred to the occipital area and associated with headaches, including facial pain
  - mid-cervical facet pain referred to the 'collar' area around the lower neck
  - lower (C5/6) cervical facet pain referred to the 'shawl' area over the shoulders
  - pain may radiate from any level down the arm in a non-radicular distribution.

Examination

- Posture—loss of cervical lordosis
- Muscles—muscle spasm or wasting, use of muscle groups to maintain posture
- Joints—range of movement, pain on movement, tender points
- Nerves—upper-limb neurological deficit, thoracic outlet syndrome.

Investigation

- X-ray—may show changes of cervical spondylosis
- MRI—exclude disc pathology and neural compromise
- Laboratory tests—exclude systemic disease.

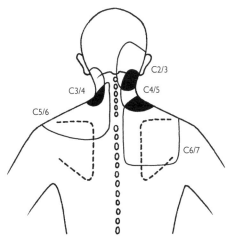

Fig. 5.3 Pain referral patterns from cervical C2/3 to C6/7 facet joint injections. Shaded areas indicate areas of pain experienced by asymptomatic volunteers after injection of facet joints C2/3 to C6/7. (Reproduced from Dwyer AB, Aprill C, Bogduk N (1990). Cervical zygapophyseal joint pain patterns. I: A study in normal volunteers. *Spine* **15**: 453–7, Lippincott-Raven Publishers.)

Medial branch block technique

Anatomy

The segmental spinal nerve passes through the intervertebral foramen before it divides into the anterior and posterior rami. The posterior ramus then divides into:

- lateral branch—supplies the paravertebral muscles and patch of skin over the neck
- medial branch—sensory supply to the facet joint.

The medial branch crosses the waist of the articular pillar in a variable position. It tends to cross at the midline at C3, but crosses at a higher level on the lower vertebrae.

The sensory innervation to the facet joint is supplied from the medial branch at the level of the joint and from a branch arising from the level above. Hence each facet joint requires a block at two cervical levels.

Patient position

Diagnostic blocks can be performed using a posterior or a lateral approach to the cervical spine. The patient needs to be positioned to obtain the optimum view of the target area. Sometimes this is not possible and the patient should be warned that on occasions the procedure cannot be completed for technical reasons.

- Prone—patient lying over a chest wedge: good access; better for lower levels.
- Lateral: comfortable; lower shoulder may obscure lower levels.
- Supine: more comfortable; suitable for upper vertebrae.

C-arm position
- C-arm and patient are positioned to obtain a clear lateral view of the target vertebra which must be 'square' with no overlap of articular pillars visible on the image (eliminate parallax) (Figs. 5.4 and 5.5).
- Use 'tunnel vision' coaxial view to approach the target point on the waist of the articular pillar.

Procedure
Lateral approach
- Obtain a clear lateral image of the cervical level to be treated.
- The target point should be in the centre of the fluoroscopy screen. This will change for each level.
- Place a marker needle on the skin over target.
- Infiltrate skin with local anaesthetic.
- Advance the needle using 'tunnel vision' to guide it until it touches the middle of the articular pillar.
- Check needle tip position in lateral and AP fluoroscopic views.
- Negative aspiration test for blood.
- Inject 0.5mL LA for diagnostic block at each level to be treated.

The C2/3 joint has a very variable nerve supply, so infiltration should be made in a line extending from the C2 mid-articular pillar target point through a point above the joint line and onto a point over the joint line. In addition, the C3 mid-articular pillar target point must be injected. This produces a 'sausage' of infiltration to cover the nerve supply at C2/3.

Posterior approach
- Obtain a clear AP image of the cervical level to be treated. The C-arm can be angled to obtain a clear image of the vertebra.
- The target is the lateral border of the 'waist' of the cervical articular pillar midway between the superior and inferior articular surfaces.
- Advance the needle using 'tunnel vision' to guide it until it touches the lateral edge of the pillar.
- Check the needle tip position in lateral and AP fluoroscopic view on the C-arm.
- Ensure that the needle tip does not lie too far anteriorly on the lateral view.

Complications
- Vasovagal syncope in up to 5% cervical procedures.
- Risk of damage to other structures is unlikely if small movements are made under fluoroscopic control with perfect alignment of the image.
- Intravascular injection is unlikely if the needle tip is accurately placed.
- Misdirection of the needle can result in placing the needle intradurally or onto the nerve root if the image is not perfectly aligned.

Assessment
- Record measures of patient's self assessment of pain, mobility, and radiation pattern before and after the diagnostic block.
- Assessments can be made immediately after the block and on subsequent days. Benefit may extend beyond the expected duration of the effect of the LA used.
- A diagnostic block can provide sustained relief for some patients.

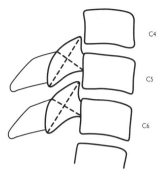

Fig. 5.4 Diagram of lateral cervical spine C-arm image showing the C5 target.

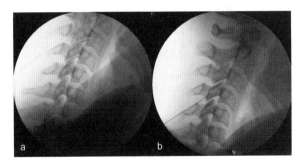

Fig. 5.5 (a) Poor image shows 'squared' C4 vertebral body but 'overlap' of facet joint lines (parallax not eliminated). (b) Good image with neither vertebra nor articular pillars showing 'overlap' (parallax eliminated). Skin marker showing the entry point for the C4 MBB.

Further reading

Bogduk N, McGuirk B (2000). *Management of Acute and Chronic Neck Pain: An Evidence-Based Approach.* Amsterdam: Elsevier.

Rathmell J (2006). *Atlas of Image-Guided Interventions.* Baltimore, MD: Lippincott–Williams & Wilkins.

Cervical facet radiofrequency denervation

Indications

Neck pain with or without radiation that can be eliminated by an LA block of the medial branch of the dorsal ramus at the levels of pain.

Patient selection

Patients who have had neck pain for at least 6 months where conservative measures have not helped. Neck pain usually arises in middle age or later, often after periods of static exertion or sudden or asymmetrical strain. It can occur in the teens and twenties as a result of trauma (e.g. whiplash type injury). Pain is often worse when bending the head backwards and to the affected side. It is also often provoked by rotation to the same side.

It is common for patients to complain of diffuse radiating pain to the trapezius that may extend to the upper arm, forearm, and fingers. This results in the pain being mistakenly interpreted as radicular. The radiation and feeling of numbness in the fingers can be very confusing when trying to interpret the source of pain. Radiation to the middle, ring, and little fingers may come from the upper cervical levels, being first reproduced and then eliminated by a medial branch block at C2/3 and C4. The lower cervical levels may produce identical radiation patterns responding to medial branch blocks at C7/T1 and T2. Previous surgery or RF neurotomy are not a contraindication to this treatment.

Clinical examination

Examination of the neck needs to be done with care and gentleness, especially in patients with whiplash trauma who suffer from severe headaches that could be provoked by the examination.

Neck movements are best tested by asking the patient to move the head themselves and to stop when it hurts. They are usually able to point to the exact area where the pain is perceived. This is much more reliable than the dermatomal area of radiation when trying to decide what levels to test. Assess reduced flexion, extension, and rotation to the sides by asking them to place the chin on the top of the shoulder. Assess side flexion by asking them to touch the shoulder with the ear; the shoulder may be raised while doing this. Provocation of pain while testing movement and where it is felt should be documented. Midline tenderness of the dorsal spines may indicate a discogenic pain component; paravertebral tenderness is usually a sign of a facet joint problem. Palpation of the occipital nerves (greater and lesser) needs to be done especially gently as this can provoke a severe headache with nausea. There is usually a clear difference in tenderness between the sides when examining a patient with unilateral neck pain with headache.

Investigations

The diagnosis is made by performing medial branch blocks using small volumes (0.5–1mL) of LA injected onto the medial branch of the dorsal ramus, taking care to avoid intravascular injections as this will give a false-negative conclusion. The easiest way to make sure of this is either to withdraw the needle a couple of millimetres while injecting or testing with contrast before injecting the LA. A positive result is 80–100% relief following injection, lasting at least for the expected duration of the LA used. In practice, there is great variation; it is common to have complete pain relief for a day or two with both bupivacaine and lidocaine. Two clearly positive blocks on two separate occasions are considered sufficient to establish the diagnosis. As each joint is supplied by two nerves, one at the same level and one from above, it is necessary to inject both. It is recommended that a minimum of three nerves (two joints), and possibly more, are injected depending on the area of pain.

Contraindications

Absolute

- Patient unwilling
- Infection at the site of treatment
- Pregnancy
- Bleeding disorders and anticoagulants

Relative contraindications

After RF denervation it is common to have an exacerbation of pain that may last from a few days to a few weeks. It is very important that the patient is aware of this and can cope; strong analgesics may be required to manage the increase in pain.

In patients with cardiac pacemakers it is good practice to involve a cardiologist with monitoring during RF denervation.

Insufficient experience when faced with patients who have advanced degenerative changes may make interpretation of the anatomy very difficult.

Consent

The patient must be aware that, after denervation:

- Despite the positive diagnostic blocks, there is no guarantee of pain relief.
- There could be pain from the procedure.
- Heavy work must be avoided during the immediate postoperative period.
- There will be some sensory loss but this usually disappears, with normal skin sensation returning in 3–6 months.

Cooperation during the procedure is imperative and communication between doctor and patient must be maintained. The procedure will require the patient to be awake and aware so that any unexpected symptom is reported immediately.

Preparation

The procedure is peformed in a room that is suitable for an aseptic procedure. It is necessary to have fluoroscopy (C-arm) facilities with a narrow
radio-translucent table (ideally 50cm wide) which allows free movement
of the C-arm so that the X-ray beam can be directed from all angles. Basic
resuscitation equipment should be available. The operator needs to be
familiar with the workings of the RF generator and the use of fluoroscopy
to obtain the best images. Lidocaine is used for skin and muscle and bupivacaine 0.5% for the target nerve prior to lesioning.

Positioning

The procedure can be performed in the prone, supine, or lateral positions.
Both the prone and the supine have some advantages and disadvantages.
The lateral position maintains the advantages of both these positions
while eliminating the disadvantages; therefore it is described in detail.
The patient lies on their side, with the side to be treated uppermost with
appropriately placed pillows for comfort. It is necessary to draw the lower
shoulder downwards in a caudal direction to obtain a good lateral image,
especially when treating the lower cervical levels (Fig. 5.6). The operator
stands behind the patient with the C-arm and the X-ray monitor on the
other side, in front of the patient. When the right side is treated the
patient lies on their left with the operator working from behind. When
the left side is treated, the patient lies on their right, with the operator
behind the patient in the same way, looking at the X-ray monitor on the
other side of the patient.

(a)

(b)

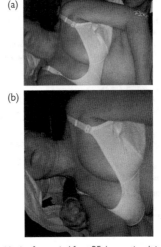

Fig. 5.6 Patient positioning for cervical facet RF denervation. It is important to push
the lower shoulder down to be able to visualize the lower neck on the lateral view.
The pillow can then be pushed down to maintain the position. Both shoulders need
to be down while working on the lower neck.

Technique

Knowledge of the anatomy of the dorsal ramus and the medial branches that supply the joints is essential. The most important anatomical features in the cervical spine are best studied by examining a skeleton. The cervical vertebrae have three clearly defined parts when seen on X-ray (Fig. 5.7). The body is in front with the articular column behind it, bordered above and below by the facet joint margins. The dorsal spine is posterior; make a note of the large posterior spine of C2 as this aids orientation. The central articular column, between the body in front and the dorsal spine behind, has a 'waist' or groove down its middle parallel to the joint margins where the nerve lies, giving off branches both cranially and caudally to supply the adjacent joint. Thus each joint obtains its nerve supply from two levels: above and below. The aim is to place the cannula parallel to these nerves and to make two or three lesions in the area close to each other to 'carpet' the nerve. An 18G cannula with a bent 10mm non-insulated tip is recommended; two adjacent lesions are usually sufficient. A finer cannula can be used, but the lesions will be smaller and more lesions will be required. A number of steps are required to perform the procedure and to get the cannula in place in the shortest possible time with absolute certainty for correct and safe placement. To get the needle parallel to the nerve, it is necessary to come from behind at about 35–45° lateral to the saggital plane (depending on the size of the neck). The correct point at which the cannula punctures the skin is crucial in achieving a satisfactory position for lesioning. If followed meticulously, the following steps will ensure satisfactory performance of this procedure.

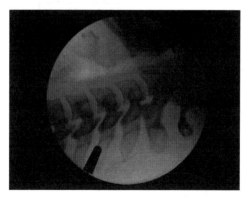

Fig. 5.7 Skin insertion point in line with the facet joints, the same distance behind the posterior margin of the articular column as the distance between the anterior and posterior borders of the articular column.

- Adjust the C-arm to obtain a 'perfect lateral' view of the target level. This implies eliminating double shadows by aligning the edges of the posterior margins of the articular column and the facet joint margins above and below.

- Deciding on where to puncture the skin requires judgment and a certain amount of 'adjustment' depending on the size of the neck. The cannula must always approach the articular column from behind and be parallel to the joint margins so that it lies in the groove or 'waist' of the articular column. Approaching from too far back will not allow the tip to cover the anterolateral aspect, close to the foramen, where the nerve emerges. If the skin puncture is not sufficiently posterior, the needle point rather than the side of the needle tip will be on the nerve. Start by making a note of the distance between the posterior border of the body of the vertebra and the posterior margins of the articular column. Mark a point on the skin that is the same distance behind the posterior margin of the articular column along a line extending backwards from the waist of the articular column (Fig. 5.7). Anaesthetize the skin, subcutaneous tissue, and muscles along the projected track towards the articular column using a 2cm needle. If the patient is large and the neck is muscular, a longer needle can be used. Care must be taken to avoid inadvertent intraspinal injection.

- The cannula is now inserted. The angle of approach is crucial as there is danger of inadvertent penetration into the gap between the laminae and entering the epidural or even intrathecal canal (with disastrous consequences). Therefore it is recommended that the cannula is inserted under real-time fluoroscopy, advancing first more superficially but no further than the anterior border of the articular column. If bone contact is not achieved, the needle is retracted and angled slightly deeper the same way until the point of the cannula makes contact with the midpoint of the articular column (Fig. 5.8). LA is injected into the muscles and when bone contact is achieved. Bupivacaine is recommended; usually 1mL is injected at bone contact but possibly a little more when final positioning is achieved, prior to lesioning.

- The curved tip can now be used to advantage. The point is turned away from the bone and the cannula is advanced while maintaining contact with bone until the point is at the posterior border of the body.

- Before the final position can be achieved, it is necessary to reposition the C-arm to an inferior oblique angle. First roll the C-arm away from yourself until you see the foramen; then tilt the C-arm inferiorly. The pedicle from the other side of the vertebrae will now look like a small ball in the middle of the body (Fig. 5.9).

- The final position can now be achieved by advancing the cannula further along the anterolateral border of the articular column, under real-time fluoroscopy, until the point is just behind the posterior border of the lower third of the foramen (Figs. 5.10 and 5.11). The tip of the cannula is rotated to point medially so that the curve of the tip lies along the anterolateral articular column.

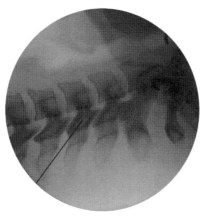

Fig. 5.8 Tip of cannula making bone contact in the middle of articular column (see Fig. 5.7).

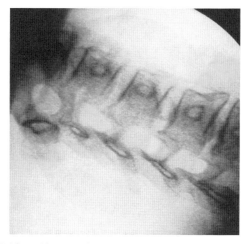

Fig. 5.9 Inferior oblique view: the opposite pedicle appears as a circular shadow in the middle of the vertebral body.

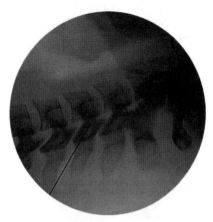

Fig. 5.10 Lateral view: cannula after being advanced up to the anterior border of the articular column (confirmed in the inferior oblique view in Fig. 5.11).

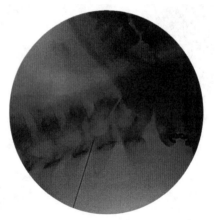

Fig. 5.11 Inferior oblique view as in Fig. 5.10: tip of cannula in place prior to lesioning (the tip does not reach the posterior border of the foramen).

Remove the stylet from the cannula and insert the RF electrode. Check that the cannula has not moved during this process. Make sure that the earth plate is in firm contact with the skin and that the RF generator indicates that connections are set. Stimulation is not necessary to confirm the correct position as this has been done reliably by different X-ray views. The first lesion can then be performed. Use the automatic mode on the RF generator, set the temperature at 85°C, and the duration to 65–70s (this allows sufficient time to reach the set temperature), and then give a 60s lesion. After this, the electrode can be moved a few millimetres superiorly using the curve to facilitate repositioning, so that it lies behind the upper third of the foramen. Carefully check the position again, making sure that the point of the cannula is clear of the posterior border before a second lesion is made. Two lesions using an 18G cannula with a 10mm tip are usually sufficient; a third lesion may be made if it is felt that full coverage of the target area was not achieved by two lesions.

The technique is the same for levels C4–C6 and will cover any variations in anatomy. At the C7 level there is greater variation in the position of the target nerve both supero-inferiorly as well as in its proximity to bone. This means that at least three lesions need to be made along the curve of the transverse process (Fig. 5.12). Since the articular column at C7 in the lateral view is shaped like a pyramid, the area along the side is usually lesioned along its entire surface from the tip downwards (Fig. 5.13). The skin puncture point for C7 is the same as that for C6. Both these levels can be treated by redirecting the cannula without pulling it right out of the skin. The muscles here are often very sensitive and require generous amounts of LA.

Great care is needed to perform RF lesioning of the third occipital nerve over the C2/3 joint safely and adequately. It is worth investing the time required to master this, as the results are most gratifying, often providing dramatic relief and a marked improvement in quality of life for patients who have suffered from severe headaches for years. What makes this level more complicated is the fact that the third occipital nerve, which leaves the C3 foramen (between C2 and C3) travelling backwards over the C2/3 facet joint, sometimes exits from the upper part of the foramen and sometimes from lower down. It is usually necessary to make four lesions along the anterolateral aspect of the articular column of C3 and on the lateral aspect of the C2/3 joint (see Fig. 5.14 (lateral views) and Fig. 5.15 (inferior oblique views)). The first lesion is made on the lower part of the C3 articular column and subsequent lesions are more cephalad; Fig. 5.14(a) and (b) show the third and fourth lesions, respectively.

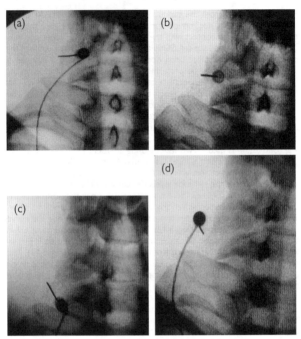

Fig. 5.12 (a)–(c) AP views of three lesions along the curve of the C7 transverse process. (d) 'Inferior tunnel' view confirming that the cannula tip is close to bone.

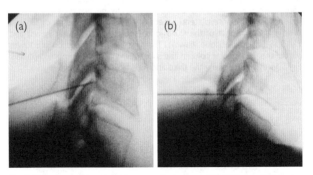

Fig. 5.13 Lesion positions from the top to the bottom of the C7 'pyramid' (lateral surface of the upper part of the transverse process) Three lesions are usually made.

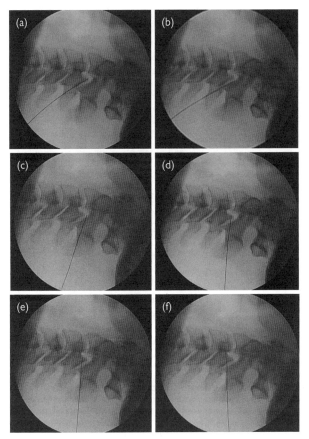

Fig. 5.14 The area to be lesioned above, on, and below the C2/3 facet joint in the lateral position.

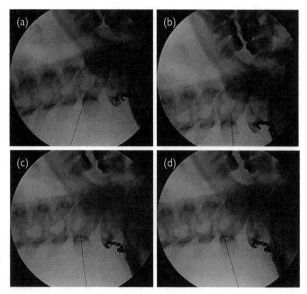

Fig. 5.15 The area to be lesioned behind the C3 foramen in the inferior oblique view. The opposite pedicle appears as a circular shadow in the middle of the vertebral bodies.

Complications

Complications are rare as long as the procedure is performed correctly with attention to detail. Infection, bleeding, and an allergic reaction to LA should be mentioned, but have not been reported. The main danger is if the RF electrode is placed wrongly because of lack of care and knowledge and is inserted too far and onto the ventral ramus. Even this will not cause damage if the patient is awake and immediately reports a burning sensation down the arm, and the operator aborts the lesion. Some radiation out to the arm during lesioning is common, and as long as the electrode position has been confirmed to be correct then there should be no problem. If the patient confirms that this is the area of pain radiation normally felt, this may allay concerns. Retracting the electrode a few millimetres until this radiation stops will result in a failure to coagulate the medial branch and produce an unsatisfactory result.

Management

Postoperative pain is the most common problem and must be managed adequately. Patients often require opioids. A week or two off work, sometimes longer, is justified, especially if their work involves significant lifting or physical exertion with the arms. Patients need to avoid exertion and take adequate analgesics. Patients should be followed up at regular intervals (usually 1, 3, 6, and 12 months). This can be done by telephone. Some or all the pain may recur after months or years. It is quite easy to confirm the cause and treat again in the same way and is usually successful.

Pearls of wisdom

- When starting, remember that the patient, who may be very frightened and tense, will often move when the needle is inserted with a loss of the 'perfect lateral' image that must be maintained during the first part of the procedure. Therefore the C-arm may need frequent adjustment. Focus your attention only on the level that is being treated, ignoring the less than perfect image at adjacent levels.
- Probably the most common cause of failure is treatment of an insufficient number of levels. It is better to treat one or more extra levels instead of trying to limit the number of levels to the minimum
- Poor patient selection using less than rigorous criteria will also result in poorer outcomes
- When the results of RF are unsatisfactory and further medial branch blocks do not eliminate the residual pain, a discogenic pain component may be a contributing factor. In these patients, a steroid epidural, when a catheter is inserted under fluoroscopy to make the injection in the area of pain and on the side of the pain, will often, but not always, provide good relief for about 3 weeks
- Another cause of persistent diffuse problems is sympathetic activity. On questioning, the patient will admit to dropping things frequently, having problems writing or doing precision work, a feeling of cold in the arm, and possibly increased sweating. The sympathetically mediated problem can be tested and often treated by an appropriate sympathetic block, preferably performed under fluoroscopy, of the lower part of the stellate ganglion at T1.

Thoracic spine interventions

T. Vasu, K.N. Shoukrey, and R. Munglani

Thoracic epidural

Introduction

- Thoracic epidural injection is a technique where drugs, including LAs and steroids, are delivered into the thoracic epidural space.
- Thoracic epidural procedures have significant risks and should only be done after simpler treatments have been used. Informed consent is essential.
- The pain clinician should not undertake these procedures without mastering lumbar procedures first. Acquisition of knowledge, skills and competencies is essential.
- Thoracic epidural injections are temporary and can relieve thoracic nerve irritation within a multimodal approach. They are not curative.

Essential equipment

Basic safety precautions should be followed as detailed in 📖 Chapter 3, p. 24. Intravenous cannula and resuscitation facilities are vital. Thoracic epidural injection requires fluoroscopy. Verbal contact should be maintained with the patient at all times; the authors are of the opinion that this reduces the risk of neurological injury.

Indications

Thoracic epidural injections are used to place drugs in the thoracic epidural space for radicular pain that is not relieved by conservative treatments. They can be:

- diagnostic—to assess the efficacy of LA and to confirm diagnosis
- therapeutic—mixture of local anaesthetic and steroid to relieve pain due to nerve irritation (e.g. disc prolapse).

Contraindications

Epidurals should not be performed for non-radicular axial pain; the evidence for this is very poor. Patient refusal, coagulopathy, local infection, and uncooperative patient are absolute contraindications.

Mechanism of action

LAs may break the pain–spasm–pain cycle and alter neuroplasticity due to modulating mechanisms. Corticosteroids are anti-inflammatory and also have LA effects; they may also wash out mediators of pain transmission. The mechanical hydrostatic effect of the injectate may also lyse adhesions.

Techniques

Position

Sitting, prone, or lateral decubitus positions can be used. Patient and technical factors usually decide the choice of the position.

Fluoroscopy

The level of the thoracic vertebra chosen should be established by AP image. 'Squaring' the vertebra by either caudal or cranial movement of the intensifier is essential so that the views show a single line for the lower margin of the vertebra. Then a caudal tilt of the image intensifier will open up the intervertebral entry space. Because of the angle of the spine at thoracic levels, the needle direction should be more acute from the skin than at the lumbar level.

If the bony landmarks are not clear, the clinician should not proceed as the risk to neurovascular structures can be catastrophic. The AP view should help identification of the vertebral anatomy so that the needle does not hit bony landmarks, and then a lateral view helps to identify the exact depth of the epidural space.

Midline or paramedian

Many clinicians prefer the midline approach for therapeutic steroid deposition, although implant procedures will need a paramedian approach (10–15°).

Translaminar technique

The skin should be cleaned and universal sterile precautions applied. Patients should understand the nature of the procedure and verbal contact must be maintained. Adequate skin infiltration with LA is needed.

Our preferred technique is an 18G Tuohy needle with loss of resistance to saline. Care should be taken when moving the needle; gradual slow movements will prevent any damage. As the needle goes through the superficial tissue layers, the C-arm is rotated to give a lateral view of the thoracic spine. This should show the vertebral foramen, especially the posterior border. The needle should be moved gently, with repeated checks of its position and depth by fluoroscopy.

As soon as the needle tip comes in contact with the posterior border of the intervertebral foramen, the clinican will feel a definite loss of resistance with saline. At this point aspiration is needed, and the position can be checked by injecting 1mL of non-ionic contrast (e.g. Omnipaque 300). This should alert the clinician to intravascular or intrathecal injection. The C-arm should be rotated to obtain an AP view and the contrast spread checked again (Fig. 6.1). Once the needle is confirmed to be in the correct position, aspiration is checked and the LA and steroid mixture are injected. We do not exceed a volume of 10mL; our preference is 4mL LA (2mL 2% lidocaine and 2mL 0.5% bupivacaine) with 2mL steroid (80mg triamcinolone acetate or, alternatively, a non-particulate steroid (e.g. dexamethasone)) and 4mL saline. If there are comorbidities or pressure symptoms, the injected volume should be reduced.

The patient should be moved to the recovery area. Vital signs should be monitored at least every 5min for 20min and then every 15min for an hour. The patient's first steps should be assisted, and they should be advised to take care when they get out of bed and walk.

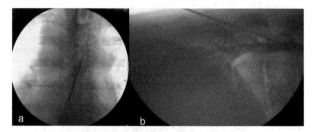

Fig. 6.1 (a) AP and (b) lateral views of the thoracic spine, showing good squared vertebrae. A paramedian entry to the epidural space with good contrast spread can be seen in both AP and lateral views.

Post-procedure care

Patients should be kept in hospital until motor power recovers fully and they pass urine. Education is vital with regard to the expectations, limitations, and side effects of the procedure. Multidisciplinary input with physiotherapy acts synergistically with the epidural. Patients should be advised about possible motor weakness. They should also be advised to avoid driving and lifting weights for 24h after the procedure. However, the opportunity should be used to advise paced walking after 24h and stretching exercises.

Patients should understand that although the LA effect will wear off in hours, the steroid could take time to work. They should be advised to keep a pain diary, including quality of life, sleep, and need for extra analgesics. We do not advise repeating the epidural more than three times a year because of the risks of long-term steroid adminstration.

Complications

Complications are rare but can be devastating. However, they can usually be avoided if appropriate precautions are taken. The artery of Adamkiewicz can originate at the mid-thoracic level and care should be taken to avoid injecting particulate steroids intravascularly (the risk is higher when using the transforaminal route). Paraplegia without any intra-procedural complaints in an awake patient due to injection into the cord has been described. In terms of risk, 40% of all chronic pain claims in the American Society of Anaesthetists (ASA) closed claims were due to epidural steroid injections (all levels). Out of 114 claims, the serious complications were infection (n = 20) and significant nerve injury (n = 28).

Reasons for failure

- Axial pain without any radiculopathy
- Multilevel spinal involvement
- Epidural fibrosis (e.g. post-surgical)
- Multiple other coexisting pain

Careful patient selection with assessment of risks versus benefits, informed consent, meticulous aseptic precautions, proper X-ray imaging in different planes, training and acquisition of competencies, and good aftercare can minimize the risks of side effects and failure of thoracic epidural injections.

Clinical pearls of wisdom

- Have all simple treatment modalities been exhausted before considering a thoracic epidural?
- Does the patient understand the technique, its limitations, and its side effects?
- Are there any bleeding or local infection risks?
- Good fluoroscopy is vital
- Is contrast spread acceptable?
- Is aspiration negative?

Further reading

Fitzgibbon DR, Posner KL, Domino KB, et al. (2004). Chronic pain management: American Society of Anesthesiologists closed claims project. *Anesthesiology* **100**: 98–105.

Tripathi M, Nath SS, Gupta RK (2005). Paraplegia after intracord injection during attempted epidural steroid injection in an awake patient. *Anesth Analg* **101**: 1209–11.

Thoracic dorsal spinal root blockade

History

Multiple level thoracic dorsal root ganglion/spinal root nerve block was historically used to provide anaesthesia for thoracic surgery. The advent of tracheal intubation and muscle relaxants have meant that it is now used to provide adjunct analgesia for operative procedures and as a diagnostic and therapeutic procedure for pain management.

Anatomy

The thoracic spinal nerves exit the intervertebral foramina just beneath the transverse process of the vertebra. After exiting the intervertebral foramen, each nerve gives off a recurrent branch that loops back through the foramen to provide innervation to the spinal ligaments, meninges, and their respective vertebrae. The thoracic spinal nerve also joins the thoracic sympathetic chain via the rami communicantes.

The thoracic spinal nerve divides into a posterior and an anterior branch. The posterior division innervates the facet joints, muscles, and skin of the back. The larger anterior division enters the subcostal groove beneath each rib to become the intercostal nerves, or the subcostal nerve in the case of the 12th intercostal nerve. These provide innervation to the skin, muscles, ribs, parietal pleura, and parietal peritoneum. Blockade of the thoracic paravertebral nerve is performed at the point where the nerve is beginning to give off its various branches, so it is possible to block the anterior division and the posterior division, as well as the recurrent and sympathetic components of each thoracic paravertebral nerve. Blockade of all these structures is generally known as a para-vertebral nerve blockade.

The pleura lie both anterior and lateral to the nerves, and this has a profound effect on the approach to these nerves. Targeted entry into the intervertebral foramina to provide specific spinal nerve blockade is not possible, as it requires a more oblique angle approach that would increase the possibility of a pneumothorax.

Indications for thoracic dorsal spinal root blockade

- Evaluation and management of pain involving chest wall, upper abdominal wall, and thoracic spine.
- Diagnostic tool when performing differential neural blockade on an anatomical basis for evaluation of chest, thoracic spine, and abdominal pain.
- Indicator of the degree of sensory and motor impairment that the patient may experience if destruction of the thoracic paravertebral nerve is being considered.
- Palliation in acute pain emergencies, including thoracic vertebral compression fracture, acute herpes zoster, and cancer pain (e.g. when waiting for pharmacology, surgery, chemotherapy, and radiotherapy to become effective).

- Treatment of post-thoracotomy pain, posterior rib fractures, and post-herpetic neuralgia.
- Destruction of the thoracic spinal nerve for the palliation of cancer pain, including invasive tumours of thoracic spine, posterior ribs, and chest/upper abdominal wall.

Technique

- General preparations for any invasive procedure are followed including assessment, preparation, and consent.
- Any form of coagulopathy is a contraindication.
- The patient is placed prone with a pillow under the lower chest to flex the thoracic spine slightly.
- Fluoroscopy is used to identify the intended level of blockade.
- The spinous process of the vertebra just above the nerve to be blocked is palpated.
- The skin at a point just below and lateral to the spinous process is prepared with antiseptic solution.
- The skin puncture site is about 4–5cm lateral to the midline or just lateral to the paravertebral edge, occasionally one may need to start slightly more lateral. (Starting more laterally increases the chances of pneumothorax.)
- A 22G 8cm needle is advanced perpendicular to skin or slightly medial, aiming to be paravertebral and inferior to the transverse process (Figs. 6.2 and 6.3(a)).
- If the needle impinges on the lateral margin of the vertebra, it should be withdrawn and directed more laterally, staying as medial as possible (i.e. paravertebral). At a depth of ~3–4cm, contact may be made with the transverse process, and then the needle is redirected inferiorly and walked off the inferior margin of the transverse process.
- After converting to a lateral X-ray view, the needle is advanced very slowly and paraesthesiae may be elicited in the distribution of the thoracic spinal nerve to be blocked or the level of the intervertebral foramina is reached (Fig. 6.3(b)). Contrast is injected in AP view under continuous fluoroscopy to rule out vascular spread and to confirm epidural spread if required (Fig. 6.4).
- If paraesthesiae have been elicited, either by the needle or contrast, and careful aspiration reveals no blood or cerebrospinal fluid, 5mL of 1.0% lidocaine or 2–2.5mL levobupivacaine 0.5% with 80mg methylprednisolone or water soluble dexamethasone 8mg is injected slowly.

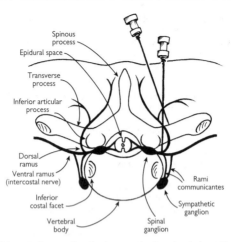

Fig. 6.2 Schematic diagram of needle placement for thoracic spinal root blockade.

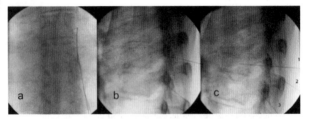

Fig. 6.3 (a) X-ray of thoracic spinal root blocks. Note how the needles pass below the transverse processes and remain parallel to the vertebral body. If the needle seems to be forced laterally, try a more lateral entry point and aim slightly medially (as seen with the lower two needles). Cephalad or caudal angulations may be required to avoid the ribs; try angling the X ray-tube caudal or cephalad to see if this helps to open the entry point between the transverse process and the rib. (b) Ideal placement of the needle on the lateral X-ray in the superior part of the intervertebral foramen. In this position eliciting painful paraesthesiae is not required and spread of injectate along the root and into the epidural space is almost certain. (c) Three needles at different depths. Needle 1 is ideal for a thoracic sympathetic block. Needle 2 is at the correct depth for a medial branch block and RF lesioning. Needle 3 has dropped below the transverse process and is lying just superior to the intervertebral foramen. Stimulation here would lead to radicular pain and chest wall movement, and conventional RF here may lead to neuritis of the spinal root.

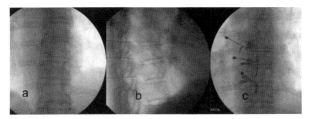

Fig. 6.4 (a) Oblique view of the thoracic spine showing the pedicle and needle entry just below the pedicle. (b) Lateral view showing the needle in position. (c) AP view showing the contrast spread.

Complications

- Pneumothorax is a possibility, given the close proximity of the pleural space. The incidence will be decreased if care is taken to keep the needle placed medially against the vertebral body and avoid it going too deeply. It certainly must not go beyond the midpoint of the vertebral body on the lateral view.
- Epidural, subdural, or subarachnoid injection or trauma to spinal cord if the needle is angled too medially.
- Exiting nerve roots can be damaged if needle placement is too aggressive.
- Infection, although uncommon, is a possibility, especially in immunocompromised patients. Early detection is crucial to avoid potentially life-threatening sequelae.

Clinical pearls of wisdom

- Neurolytic block with small quantities of 6% aqueous phenol or in glycerine 1–5mL or by cryoneurolysis or pulsed RF lesioning (40 degrees C for 6min) may provide longer-term relief for patients suffering from post-thoracotomy and cancer-related pain who have not responded to conservative treatments.
- Occasionally the position of the rib can make access difficult. Initially aiming the needle tip at the top or middle of the transverse process when penetrating the skin (and staying paravertebral but then aiming caudad) may help.
- Avoid going laterally or beyond the midpoint of the vertebral body on the lateral view to avoid penetrating the pleura (see Fig. 6.3(c) and Chapter 11, p. 189).

Thoracic facet joint medial branch blockade

Anatomy

The thoracic facet joints are paired synovial joints formed by the articulation of the superior and inferior articular facets of adjacent vertebrae. They are true joints in that they are lined with synovium and possess a true joint capsule that is richly innervated and so can become a pain generator.

The poor localization of facet joint pain is explained in part by the pattern of overlapping of the sensory innervation of these joints and their close proximity to one another. The posterior rami of a nerve root diverge from the spine at the intervertebral foramen and pass dorsally and caudally through the intertransverse ligament where they divide into medial, lateral, and intermediate branches. The medial branch crosses over the top of the transverse process at a variable point lateral to the point at which the transverse process meets the vertebra. The nerve then travels medially and inferiorly across the surface of the transverse process to innervate the facet joint (Fig. 6.5). The medial branch supplies the lower pole of the facet joint at its own level and the upper pole of the facet joint below. Therefore each facet joint receives its innervation from a medial branch nerve of two posterior primary rami. One branch arises from the nerve at the same level as the joint, and the other from the segmental level above. This explains why the dorsal nerve from the vertebra above the affected level must often also be blocked to provide complete pain relief.

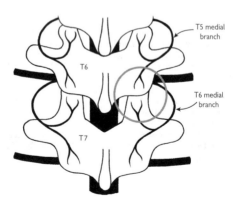

Fig. 6.5 Schematic representation of path of the thoracic medial branches at the T5–T7 levels. The medial branches of T5/T6 are labelled, note how they enter on to the superior surface of the transverse process more laterally than in the lumbar region. The thoracic facet joint is circled.

Presentation of thoracic facet syndrome

Thoracic facet joint syndrome results from a sudden twisting motion, twisting when lifting overhead, or an unguarded rotating motion of the thoracic spine. The resultant pain may be mild, dull, and aching, with radiation encircling the chest, or it may be sharp pleuritic-type pain that can affect lung functional vital capacity and overwhelm the patient. There is usually decreased motion in the portion of the spine involved. Examination of the patient may reveal a loss of the thoracic curve or muscle spasms, causing localized scoliosis.

Indications

There is no known anatomical, imaging, or histopathological standard for identifying a painful facet joint. One must clinically evaluate patients with suspected facet-related pain, select those with symptomatic facets, and then decide at which levels to make the injections. Facet-induced pain is currently a diagnosis of exclusion supported by abolition of pain after injection of LA into the joint or onto the two medial branch nerves supplying the joint.

The major indications for facet joint injection include the following.
- Focal tenderness over a facet joint and referred pain that may be vague and referred widely (Fig. 6.6).
- Chronic thoracic pain with or without radiation.
- In our experience the presentation may include abdominal pain.

Inclusion criteria for thoracic facet or medial branch injections are as follows.
- Pain for at least 6 months with other causes having been excluded by MRI scans and possibly blood tests, CT scans, X-rays, bone scans, and tests for other thoracic and abdominal causes. Progressive and/or night pain should prompt a careful search for other causes, especially in those with a history of smoking.
- Non-specific rather than radicular pain (Fig. 6.6).
- Lack of a neurological deficit, with no radicular symptoms or pain that involves predominantly the upper back and extremities.
- Failed conservative management including physical therapy, chiro-practic manipulation, exercises, drug therapy, and bed rest.

Contraindications

Facet blocks should not be performed in patients with:
- systemic infection
- infection at the site of injection
- allergies to the medication being injected
- coagulopathy (relative contraindication).

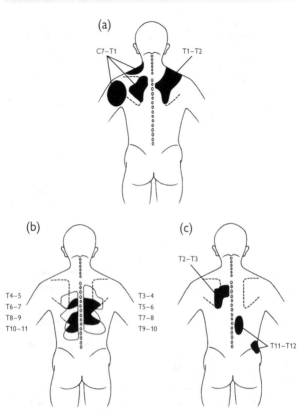

Fig. 6.6 Typical patterns of thoracic facet joint pain.

Procedure
The standard local protocol for aseptic technique, LA, and sedation should be used if required.

Positioning
- Prone
- Pillows placed under the chest to allow the thoracic spine to be moderately flexed without causing discomfort to the patient

Intra-articular technique
We do not recommend intra-articular facet joint blocks as routine. The joint space is narrow and difficult to access. Occasionally the need arises

for a specific intra-articular injection as a diagnostic manoeuvre to prove that a specific facet joint is the source of pain.

- Patient is prone with fluoroscopy.
- The joint to be blocked is identified by counting the ribs from T1 caudad and from T12 cephalad.
- The C-arm is tilted caudally. This allows identification and visualization of the articular pillars of the respective vertebrae and the adjacent facet joints.
- The steep angle of the thoracic facet joints means that the skin entry point may need to overlie the pedicle one or two segments caudad.
- After sterile preparation and draping, LA is injected into the skin and tissues along the needle path.
- A 22G 10cm spinal needle is directed steeply cephalad towards the joint. The needle is then advanced into the joint using a combination of antero-posterior and lateral fluoroscopic images (Fig. 6.7).
- The stylet is removed and, if the aspiration test is negative, the joint is injected.
- Thoracic facet joints are very small and can hold only 0.4–0.6mL of injectate. Therefore the mixture of contrast, LA, and steroid should not exceed the joint volume. Additional solution is often injected peri-articularly for therapeutic purposes.

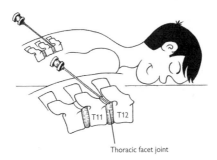

Thoracic facet joint

Fig. 6.7 Diagram illustrating needle entry point.

Medial branch technique

This technique is useful in the diagnosis of pain mediated by thoracic medial braches, usually arising from facet joints. A prognostic medial branch block is useful for predicting whether RF lesioning of the affected joint(s) may provide long-lasting relief of pain originating from the facet joints. It is important to note the variability in the medial branch path as previously explained (Fig 6.5).

- The patient is prone with fluoroscopy.
- After squaring the vertebral endplates, the C-arm is rotated obliquely to identify and visualize the junction of the transverse process and vertebra at the level to be blocked
- A 22G 10cm spinal needle is inserted using an aseptic technique, LA, and sedation as required.
- The needle is then repositioned under fluoroscopic guidance until it is visualized pointing directly towards a lateral point on the transverse process (Fig. 6.8(a)). Needle placement is confirmed by fluoroscopy. The medial branch crosses the transverse process. Some authorities suggest infiltration at the superior lateral margin of the transverse process (Fig. 6.5). In our experience, probing anywhere on the middle third of the posterior aspect transverse process is satisfactory. The superior surface of the transverse process is then infiltrated with up to 1.5mL of LA with or without steroid after gentle aspiration of the needle checking for blood or CSF.

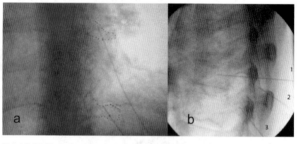

Fig. 6.8 (a) Blockade of the thoracic medial branch. We find that this is conveniently achieved by placing the needle on the middle third of the transverse process. The outline of the latter has been marked with small dots. In our experience, the tip of the transverse process may not be clearly visible, making it difficult to block the medial branch there (Fig. 6.5). With careful X-ray adjustment, the 'Scotty dog' appearance can be seen just as in the lumbar region, particularly in the lower thoracic region. This positioning is also ideal for thoracic medial branch denervation. We prefer to place the RF needle parallel to the surface of the middle third of the transverse process. Choice of this site means that the medial branch is effectively cauterized regardless of where it passes on the transverse process. Some authorities suggest the lesion is made at the superior lateral margin of the transverse process (Figs. 6.5 and 6.9) where the medial branch tends to cross onto the posterior aspect of the transverse process. This much more lateral approach often does not reveal the greatest sensitivity, and our concern is that a more medial crossing of the nerve may be missed by the RF probe. (b) Lateral view of the thoracic spine. Three needles are at different depths. Needle 1 is ideal for a thoracic sympathetic block. Needle 2 is at the correct depth for a medial branch block and RF lesioning although, ideally, it should be 'flatter', i.e. parallel to the surface of the transverse process to ensure maximum contact. Needle 3 has dropped below the transverse process and is lying just superior to the intervertebral foramina. Stimulation here may lead to radicular pain and chest wall movement; conventional RF here may lead to neuritis of the spinal root.

RF lesioning of the medial branch of the primary posterior rami

RF lesioning of the thoracic facet joints is a reasonable next step for patients with chronic dorsal spine pain that is temporarily relieved by LA block of either the affected facet joints directly, or the medial branch. Some authors suggest that two comparative blocks should be performed to rule out false positives prior to considering RF lesioning.

- The patient is prone with fluoroscopy
- After squaring the vertebral endplates, the C-arm is rotated obliquely to identify and visualize the junction of the transverse process and vertebra at the level to be blocked
- After sterile preparation, LA, and sedation, the RF cannula is directed using lateral and AP fluoroscopy (as described for medial branch block)
- The exposed tip of the RF probe should rest parallel against the bone of the transverse process in the middle third (Fig. 6.8(a)). To achieve maximum lesion size the tip of the RF needle should be parallel rather than perpendicular to the bony surface of the transverse process. It is important to remember that the medial branch position varies more in the thoracic area than in the lumbar region
- After confirmation of proper needle placement, stimulation at 50 Hz is carried out with the patient reporting stimulation between 0.1 and 0.5V; this may reproduce the patient's pain pattern. Motor stimulation of the RF needle at 2–3V and 2Hz is performed to exclude stimulation at the chest or thoracic wall in a segmental distribution. If motor stimulation occurs, the needle may be too close to the thoracic nerve root
- After injection of LA, an RF lesion is made either at 80–90°C for 60–90s or by multiple 180s 60°C lesions using a Thoracool® RF system
- The needle is then repositioned 2–3mm medially or laterally, and second and subsequent lesions are performed
- Some advocate the use of the cooled RF system developed by Baylis, which gives a larger lesion and probably a better result (Fig. 6.9).

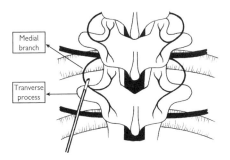

Fig. 6.9 Thoracic medial branch denervation performed at the point were the medial branch begins to cross the transverse process. We find that a conventional RF probe gives a less consistent outcome, and also that the lateral third of the transverse process is often difficult to visualize. However, the Thoracool® system developed by Baylis may offer significant advantages as the lesion size may be more than three times larger in each dimension, essentially giving a much larger and therefore more effective lesion. Here the Thoracool® probe has been placed more laterally than in Fig. 6.8(a).

Complications

The proximity to the spinal cord and exiting nerve roots makes it imperative that these procedures are only carried out by those well versed in regional anatomy and experienced in performing interventional pain management techniques.

Complications following facet blocks are rare, but include the following.

- Infection.
- Allergic reaction to the drugs used.
- Transient increase in thoracic pain.
- Pneumothorax is possible, given the proximity of the pleural space.
- Epidural, subdural, or subarachnoid injection and trauma to the spinal cord may result if the needle is placed too medial.
- Trauma to the nerve roots may result if the needle is placed too deep between the transverse processes (Fig. 6.8(b)).
- Facet joint rupture is possible with the intra-articular approach.

Clinical pearls

- Avoid intra-articular thoracic facet joint blockade as this may be associated with an increase the rate of complications.
- RF lesioning of the thoracic facets using the medial branch approach is the preferred technique for providing long-lasting relief from pain and disability associated with thoracic facet joint syndrome.
- The risks of neuritis, subarachnoid injection, and pneumothorax are minimal if the needle is kept in the medial third of the transverse process (Fig. 6.8(b)) or in the superolateral position (Fig. 6.9) whilst performing either medial branch blocks or RF lesioning. Incremental corrections and measured advancement of the needle with frequent imaging are required to ensure accuracy of needle placement.

Disc procedures

S. Gupta, A.R. Cooper, R.D. Searle, and K. Simpson

Lumbar discography

Introduction

Discogenic pain is a common cause of low back pain (LBP) in patients less than 50 years old. Patients complain of aching LBP referred to the back of the thigh. Pain is commonly above the knee joint, but it can sometimes refer to calf muscles. Discogenic pain increases on straining, coughing, and bending forwards. An MRI scan can show disc degeneration, disc bulging, annular tear, and/or disc prolapse; this may be associated with radicular pain. The lumbar intervertebral disc is innervated and provocative discography attempts to identify the painful disc.

Asepsis and antibiotic prophylaxis

Discography should be performed under strict aseptic conditions using a needle-through-needle technique. In our opinion antibiotic prophylaxis to prevent discitis can be better achieved by intradiscal antibiotic mixed with contrast (e.g. 10mg/mL cefuroxime or 10mg/mL clindamycin). However, the choice of antibiotic varies and depends on local infection control guidelines.

Procedure

The patient is positioned prone and an AP fluoroscopic view is used to identify the chosen level(s). Discography is commonly performed at three levels to obtain the most useful information. Vertebral endplates are squared by caudal or cephalic tilt of the C-arm. The superior articular process (SAP) is brought to the centre of the vertebral body by right or left oblique rotation of the C-arm. The needle entry point is just in front of the SAP in the centre of the disc; a gun-barrel approach is used.

The patient is awake or lightly sedated. A single- or double-needle technique can be used; a double-needle technique is preferred as this probably reduces the risk of infection. A 150mm 22G or 25G needle can be used for the single-needle technique. A 90mm 18G or 22G spinal needle and a companion 150mm 22G or 25G needle are used for the double-needle technique. The needle tip should not be touched or handled by the gloved hand; use sterile gauze if the tip of the needle needs bending.

Use normal 3D principles to navigate the needle. The direction of the needle is judged in the AP or oblique view; the depth is judged in the lateral view. It is essential to re-check the direction of the needle in the AP or oblique view. Once the needle is in the centre of the disc in the lateral view, obtain an AP view to confirm that the tip of the needle is in the area corresponding to the middle third of the ipsilateral hemi-vertebra (Fig. 7.1). Needles should be placed in all the discs under investigation before injecting anything. Once the needle positions are confirmed, inject contrast with antibiotics. When performing discography it is better to inject the disc least likely to be painful first. Stop injecting the contrast if concordant pain is reproduced or the contrast is seen leaking out of the disc after 2.5mL is injected. Repeat the same process at all levels and assess the response.

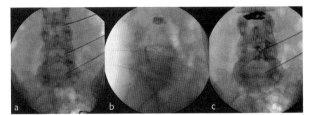

Fig. 7.1 (a) AP view—the tips of the needles can be seen in the area of the middle third of the ipsilateral hemivertebra. (b) On injecting contrast at L3/4 a nucleogram was obtained; the patient did not complain of concordant pain. At L4/5 the contrast can be seen leaking out of the disc into the anterior epidural space; the patient complained of concordant pain. (c) AP view of the same patient as in (b) with the contrast spread at L4/5.

Ideally, a pressure-monitoring device should be used. If the intradiscal pressure is monitored, four classes of discs can be identified using pounds per square inch (psi) as follows:
- discs that are painful at <15psi above opening pressure
- discs that are painful at 15–50psi above opening pressure
- discs that are painful at >50psi above opening pressure
- disc that are not painful even at pressures >50psi.

Indviduals with discs which appear normal and asymptomatic individuals do not normally complain of pain on provocation discography at intradiscal pressures <15psi. If a disc is painful <15psi, it is considered positive. If a disc is painful between 15 and 50psi, it may or may not be positive. If a disc is painful at >50psi, this is not significant.
- See Fig. 1.5: the patient is prone. AP view with the lower vertebral endplate of L4 squared off. For lower lumbar levels a cephalic tilt and for upper lumbar levels a caudal tilt of the C-arm is necessary to square the vertebral end plates.
- See Fig. 1.4(a): right oblique view with the SAP in the middle of the vertebral body. The needle is seen in front of the SAP and in the direction of the L4/5 disc.
- See Fig. 1.4(b): Lateral view—the tips of the needles can be seen in the centre of the disc spaces.

Interpretation

Concordant pain reproduced at one level and no pain or non-concordant pain at the other two levels is strongly suggestive of discogenic pain at one level. Concordant pain reproduced at two levels with no pain or non-concordant pain at one level is suggestive of discogenic pain. Pain reproduced at all three levels means that the test is inconclusive. Axial CT scanning after discography may be performed to obtain information about the internal structure of the discs studied (CT discography).

Complications

- Bleeding
- Infection
- Nerve root injury
- Discitis (significantly reduced with the use of intradiscal antibiotics)
- Headache
- Paraplegia
- Bowel perforation.

Practical tips

Bending the distal 1–2cm of the needle by about 5–10° can help to navigate the needle, especially at the L5/S1 level.

Further reading

Bogduk N (ed) (2004). Lumbar disc stimulation. In: *Practice Guidelines: Spinal Diagnostic and Treatment Procedures*, pp.20–46. San Francisco, CA: ISIS.

Bogduk N, Tynan W, Wilson AS (1981). The nerve supply to the human lumbar intervertebral discs. *J Anat* **132**: 39–56.

Derby R, Howard MW, Grant JM, *et al.* (1999). The ability of pressure-controlled discography to predict surgical and nonsurgical outcomes. *Spine* **24**: 364–72.

Groen G, Baljet B, Drukker J (1990). Nerves and nerve plexuses of the human vertebral colums. *Am J Anat* **188**: 282–96.

Klessig HT, Showsh SA, Sekorski A. The use of intradiscal antibiotics for discography: an *in vitro* study of gentamycin, cefazolin and clindamycin. *Spine* **28**: 1735–8.

Cervical discography

Introduction

Neck pain is a common complaint that affects most people at some time in their life. Most cases resolve spontaneously, but some people develop chronic neck pain.

Cervical discography or provocative discography is used in the investigation of chronic axial neck pain to establish if a particular disc or discs are the source of pain. This involves a percutaneous injection of radio-opaque contrast into the centre of a disc to elicit concordant pain. It is not commonly performed, and it usually follows clinical examination, X-rays, CT, or MRI. It is often used after other sources of neck pain, such as facet joints, have been excluded. It is an invasive procedure that should only be undertaken by practitioners experienced in cervical spine imaging and procedures as the margin for error is very low and there are many possible serious consequences. Cervical discography is the only investigation that actively determines whether the disc is a pain generator. It can be helpful in selecting patients for fusion surgery.

Indications

- Diagnosis of discogenic pain
- Consideration for spinal fusion

Contraindications

- Local or generalized infection
- Allergy to radio-opaque contrast
- Cord compression and cervical myelopathy
- Spinal canal stenosis

Procedure

- A skilled operator familiar with spinal radiological anatomy using a strict aseptic technique is essential.
- Intradiscal antibiotics are given to prevent disc infection. We recommend using a non-ionic contrast medium with 10mg/mL of cefuroxime or clindamycin or 2mg/mL of gentamycin to stimulate the disc. However, the choice of antibiotic may vary with local infection control guidelines.
- The patient should be supine with the neck extended and the skin over the anterolateral area of the neck prepared using antiseptic solution.
- The patient should be awake and not sedated, with verbal contact maintained throughout the procedure.
- A right paratracheal approach is used with AP fluoroscopy to identify the vertebral bodies. The C-arm is rotated obliquely towards the right side and slightly caudally to maximally open up and view the disc spaces with the uncovertebral junction clearly identified.
- The carotid artery is retracted posterolaterally.

- A needle-through-needle technique is used (18G introducer and 22G spinal needle) after skin infiltration with LA as far as bone before carefully advancing the needle between the trachea and the sternomastoid, avoiding the vascular structures.
- Curved tips help in steering the needle towards the centre of the disc after walking it off the lower vertebral body.
- AP and lateral views are used to target the needle pathway into the centre of the disc (Fig. 7.2). Increased resistance is felt as the disc annulus is entered.
- This procedure is repeated for at least two other discs and the position of the needles is checked.
- Contrast with antibiotic is injected in a small volume up to a maximum of 0.5mL and the patient's response is noted. It is vital to watch carefully for flow of contrast into the epidural space.
- Only gentle pressure should be used. There is little cervical epidural space which, if already compromised by protruding disc material, can be further narrowed with neurological consequences.
- Pain response is either concordant or non-concordant. A positive response is usually associated with a pain score >7/10, but wide variations are seen. Other observations, such as vocalization, facial grimacing, and withdrawal reactions, should be considered in assessing the response to disc stimulation at each level tested.
- LA can be injected into a painful disc to improve patient comfort after the antibiotic has been administered (this is usually painful).
- Control discs are necessary to compare with the expected abnormal disc.
- Annular pathology can be observed on a post-discography CT scan. There is a window of 4h to do this before the injected contrast material disappears.
- Flare-up of neck pain is usually experienced immediately after the procedure and can persist from a few days to more than a week. Analgesics are required. Patients are usually reviewed within 2 weeks.

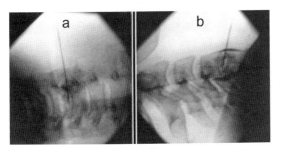

Fig. 7.2 (a) AP and (b) lateral views showing the needle positioned in the centre of disc.

Complications

- Infection—discitis, abscess (0.1–0.2%)
- Neurological injury (e.g. cord injection)
- Haematoma
- Disc herniation
- Injury to neck soft tissue structures

Discography is a controversial investigation that can be useful in some carefully selected patients where there is persistent neck pain in the absence of abnormalities. It can be useful prior to consideration of cervical fusion surgery and may improve outcomes.

Discography must be interpreted with care as many of those with positive discography improve without surgery. Those with psychological issues may report inconsistent pain during discography injection of the contrast medium. Discography remains the only useful objective predictive test for disc-mediated pain.

Further reading

Bogduk N (ed) (2004). Lumbar disc stimulation. In: *Practice Guidelines: Spinal Diagnostic and Treatment Procedures*, pp.20–46. San Francisco, CA: ISIS.

Bogduk N, Tynan W, Wilson AS (1981). The nerve supply to the human lumbar intervertebral discs. *J Anat* **132**: 39–56.

Derby R, Howard MW, Grant JM, et al. (1999). The ability of pressure-controlled discography to predict surgical and nonsurgical outcomes. *Spine* **24**: 364–72.

Groen G, Baljet B, Drukker J (1990). Nerves and nerve plexuses of the human vertebral colums. *Am J Anat* **188**: 282–96.

Klessig HT, Showsh SA, Sekorski A. The use of intradiscal antibiotics for discography: an *in vitro* study of gentamycin, cefazolin and clindamycin. *Spine* **28**: 1735–8.

Percutaneous disc decompression

Introduction

Percutaneous disc decompression (PDD) using coblation, also called nucleoplasty, is a minimally invasive technique to decompress small disc protrusions. Coblation removes disc material by using RF energy to excite electrolytes, creating a plasma field that breaks down molecular bonds and thus dissolves disc tissue. In addition to the physical removal of disc material, coblation produces biochemical changes that may reduce discogenic pain. Alterations in interleukin levels are associated with a repair response within the disc. In May 2006 the National Institute for Health and Clinical Excellence (NICE) in the UK approved PDD and produced guidance on using coblation.

Indications

Back and leg pain caused by contained herniated discs that have failed to respond to conservative management (e.g. steroid injection, physical therapy).
- Radicular pain:
  - small (<6mm) contained disc protrusion
  - disc height >50%.
- Axial back pain (little supporting evidence):
  - small contained disc protrusion
  - disc height >75%
  - low-volume low-pressure-sensitive disc.

Contraindications

- Local or systemic infection.
- Bleeding diathesis or anticoagulation.
- Progressive neurological deficit.
- Spinal fracture or tumour.
- Moderate to severe spinal stenosis.
- Severe disc degeneration (>50% loss of disc height).
- Disc hernia more than a third of the sagittal diameter of the spinal canal.

Technique

Preparation

- Consent should include discussion of the likely success rate and potential complications. All patients must be warned about the risk of discitis. All patients should have received or have had access to the relevant documents giving guidance about PDD for patients.
- Position the patient prone on a radiolucent table with a pillow under the abdomen. It is important before commencing to ensure that it is possible to obtain clear views of the target disc(s); this often requires oblique C-arm positions. The L5/S1 disc is often the most difficult to image. A fluoroscopic C-arm with sterile covers is needed.
- Equipment should include a PDD Perc DC SpineWand with introducer needle, patient cable, and coblation controller. A suitable contrast medium with antibiotics is needed if performing discography.

- Strict asepsis is essential, including sterile skin preparation, surgical drapes, surgical mask, gown, gloves, and hat.
- Introduction of the needle can be stimulating and sedation may be used. The plasma disc extraction itself is not usually painful. Verbal contact with the patient must be maintained.

Lumbar disc decompression

- An AP image of the spine should be obtained to identify the target disc.
- The X-ray beam should be rotated to view the disc from its postero-lateral aspect. The SAP of the appropriate vertebra (e.g. L5 SAP for L4/5 disc PDD) should be centred over the target disc.
- The target point lies just lateral to the lateral margin of the SAP, equidistant between the endplates of the two vertebral bodies. The skin and subcutaneous tissues over this point are infiltrated with local anaesthetic (Fig. 1.6).
- A small incision is made and the introducer needle is then advanced carefully down in line with the X-ray beam using the gun-barrel approach.
- The introducer needle can then be advanced into the disc. AP and lateral X-rays are needed to confirm the needle position.
- Take precautions to ensure a central disc entry on a lateral fluoroscopic view to avoid the wand touching the periostium.
- The wand is then inserted through the needle and its position checked on AP and lateral views (Fig. 7.3). The final image should be stored.
- The controller is set at power level 2 and the foot pedal used to control the coblation.
- Six passes are made using the wand. The wand is rotated with each pass to create a new channel in the disc material. Coblation should only occur when advancing the wand into the disc (over 5s). Care should be taken not to coblate where the wand could damage a nerve root. If the patient complains of radicular pain, coblation must be stopped. Remember not to keep the pedal on when withdrawing the wand into the needle as this can irritate the nerve root.
- Remove the introducer and wand.
- A new needle is needed for each disc to be treated.

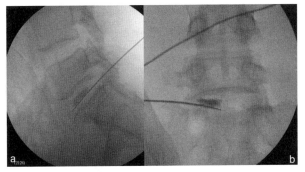

Fig. 7.3 (a) AP and (b) lateral X-ray views showing the wand in place.

Disc Dekompressor

Patient selection and needle placement are similar to PDD. The Disc Dekompressor developed by Stryker uses an Archimedes pump principle to extract nucleus pulposus. This extraction reduces intradiscal pressure and pressure on the surrounding area, providing pain relief.

Aftercare

Patients are advised to avoid positions that place pressure on the disc (e.g. sitting or standing for long periods) for 5 days following the procedure. After this, physiotherapy should be instituted to prevent problems with muscular spasm and build core stability and strength. Symptoms of radicular pain may take up to 2 weeks to resolve. Ideally pre- and post-procedure pain, function, and medication use should be recorded. It is important to obtain objective evidence of the effects of PDD.

Complications

- 76% short-term (<2 weeks) increase in pain at needle insertion point.
- 26% new numbness and tingling 24h after procedure, falling to 15% at 2 weeks.
- 4% increased intensity of pre-procedural back pain.
- Infectious discitis: rare but reported examples; exact incidence unknown. It is known that the incidence of discitis associated with discography is 0–1.3% per disc.
- Adverse events are uncommon; there are no reports in the literature of serious complications. Histological studies in animals suggest that nucleoplasty produces little local trauma. Bleeding and nerve damage are theoretical complications.

Further reading

Bhagia SM, Slipman CW, Nirschl M, *et al.* (2006). Side effects and complications after percutaneous disc decompression using coblation technology. *Am J Phys Med Rehabil* **85**: 6–13.

Bonaldi G, Baruzzi F, Facchinetti A, Facchinetti P, Lunghi S (2006). Plasma radiofrequency-based diskectomyfor treatment of cervical herniated nucleus pulposus: feasibility, safety, and preliminary clinical results. *Am J Neuroradiol* **27**: 2104–11.

Manchikanti L, Derby R, Benyamin RM, Helm S, Hirsch JA (2009). A systematic review of mechanical lumbar disc decompression with nucleoplasty. *Pain Physician* **12**: 561–72.

NICE (2006). *Percutaneous Disc Decompression Using Coblation for Lower Back Pain.* Available online at: http://www.nice.org.uk/nicemedia/pdf/ip/IPG173guidance.pdf.

Pobiel RS, Schellhas KP, Pollei SR, Johnson BA, Golden MJ, Eklund JA (2006). Diskography: infectious complications from a series of 12,634 cases. *Am j Neuroradiol* **27**: 1930–2.

Biaculoplasty for lumbar discogenic pain

Introduction

Biaculoplasty is a recently introduced minimally invasive transdiscal RF technique for treatment of LBP. Biaculoplasty uses two internally water-cooled RF probes to lesion nociceptors in the intervertebral disc. The bilateral approach is intended to facilitate controlled lesioning between the electrodes in the disc. The successful use of this therapy for severe axial LBP was reported in 2007. Further studies are ongoing and outcomes will not be discussed further.

Lumbar discogenic pain is predominantly LBP arising from intervertebral discs that have internal disc disruption (IDD) without signs of disc protrusions. A prevalence of 30–50% in patients with LBP has been reported. The disc to be treated should have been established as the source of the pain by provocative discography as clinical examination is unreliable even when supplemented with radiological examinations.

Factors involved in discogenic pain include:
- irritation of nerve endings in the outer third of the annulus
- sensitization of nociceptors in chronic discogenic pain
- ingrowth of granulation tissue and small unmyelinated nerve fibres.

Many attempts at heating the disc have been tried over the years including RF to the nucleus, direct thermal heating coils such as IDET, and the Disctrode using RF across the posterior annulus through a single curved electrode.

Biaculoplasty concentrates RF current between two straight electrodes across the posterior annulus of the disc. The electrodes are internally cooled, allowing a large deep area of controlled even heating and denervation (Fig. 7.4). There are peripheral temperature sensors at both the electrode tip and the periphery of the heating zone to ensure that the peripheral compartment temperature does not rise above 39°C; this prevents damage to the nerve root.

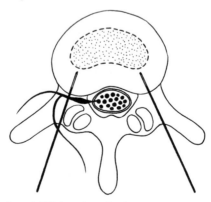

Fig. 7.4 Bipolar cooled RF electrodes in place for biaculoplasty.

Benefits of biaculoplasty

- Technically easier to perform than other methods used to date.
- Straightforward placement of electrodes into the outer annulus.
- Post-procedural pain is less than with other techniques as artificial concentric fissures caused by attempts to pass electrodes along the annulus to cover the tear being treated are avoided.

Patient selection

- Discogenic pain with positive diagnosis from discography
- Failed conservative therapy
- Axial LBP more than referred leg pain
- Abnormal disc morphology
- Disc height maintained as >50% normal
- No sequestrated or extruded disc herniation
- No segmental instability
- Single-level disc degeneration

Less likely to benefit

- Overweight
- Significant secondary gain issues
- Significant psychological issues
- Multilevel degenerative disc disease

Technique

- Place the patient prone with pillows under the abdomen to reduce lumbar lordosis.
- Strict aseptic technique.
- Maintain verbal contact with patient. Do not anaesthetize or over-sedate them.
- Good radiological views employing correct use of C-arm fluoroscopy are essential to identify target structures.
- Identify the level of disc to be treated. Square the endplates by rotating the beam caudal-cranially or cranial-caudally as appropriate to the level being treated.
- Anaesthetize the skin entry point with LA. The facet joint line should be approximately one-third of the way along the lower end plate line.
- Advance the introducer in tunnel vision or using the line-of-sight approach. Stay close to the SAP and midway between the end plate lines. Avoid contact with the nerve root that lies more superio-laterally. Disc entry is felt as an increase in resistance to the passage of the introducer.
- Repeat this on the opposite side and check a lateral view to determine the depth of entry of the probe into the disc (Fig. 7.5(a)). This should be at the junction between the posterior third and the anterior two-thirds. The temperature sensors should be visible.
- Finally, check an AP view to ensure that electrode tips do not project beyond the medial edge of the interfacet joint line and are away from the vertebral end plates (Fig. 7.5(b)).

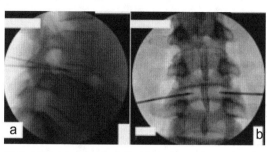

Fig. 7.5 Radiological target location for biaculoplasty.

Only when correct positioning is established and the tissue impedance is <400Ω should the treatment begin. The operator should be experienced in using the Baylis cooled RF generator. The cooled RF program ensures that gradual step-up RF heating achieves intradiscal temperatures of ~60–65°C across the posterior annulus using a validated algorithm built into the program. The circulated sterile water used in cooling the electrode tips does not come into contact with the patient's tissues; it is contained within the system tubing.

At the end of the procedure prophylactic intradiscal antibiotics are administered according to local guidelines as the probes are removed. No earth plate is used, as it is a bipolar technique.

After the procedure patients are observed for an hour in a recovery area to ensure that there is no leg weakness. Dressings are removed on the following day. Patients are advised to avoid swimming or bathing for a few days to reduce risk of infection. Showering is permitted the following day. Excessive bending, twisting, or straining should be avoided for several weeks until the disc is healed. Usually, only simple oral analgesics are required for a few days. Patients are reviewed at 2 weeks; any concerns about persistent increasing back pain or fever should alert the treating team to exclude disc infection or epidural abscess. Post-procedural physiotherapy should be encouraged to improve and maintain core stability.

Complications

- Nerve trauma
- Infection
- Haematoma
- Flare-up of pain.

Large randomized controlled trials are required to evaluate the place of this intuitively attractive technique in interventional pain practice.

Further reading

Kapural L, Mekhail N (2007). Novel intradiscal biacuplasty (IDB) for the treatment of lumbar discogenic pain. *Pain Pract* **7**: 130–4.

Vertebroplasty and kyphoplasty

P. Sinha and J. Timothy

Osteoporosis

Introduction

The World Health Organization (WHO) defines osteoporosis on the basis of bone mineral density (BMD) which is measured by dual-energy X-ray absorptiometry (DEXA). Osteoporosis is defined as a BMD that is 2.5 SD below the mean BMD of the young adult population for that gender at their peak bone mass (T-score –2.5 or lower). Clinically, osteoporosis is defined as a progressive systemic skeletal disorder characterized by low bone mass and micro-architectural deterioration in bone tissue, resulting in increased bone fragility and susceptibility to fractures. Osteoporosis affects both sexes but 80% of patients are women as the rate of bone loss increases with decrease in oestrogen production post-menopause.

Osteoporotic fractures can occur anywhere in the skeleton. The most common sites are the distal forearm, proximal femur, lower thoracic and lumbar vertebrae, and humerus. The occurrence of an osteoporotic fracture increases the risk of subsequent fractures. Within 1 year of sustaining a vertebral fracture, one in five women will experience another fracture. This is often referred to as the fracture cascade. It is estimated that there are 180,000 osteoporosis-related symptomatic fractures in England and Wales annually; 70,000 are hip fractures, 25,000 are clinical vertebral fractures, and 41,000 are wrist fractures. In the UK, the average length of hospital stay following a vertebral fracture is 19.3 days. Hospital and outpatient cost of each vertebral fracture is estimated to be £1706. There is a 4.4-fold increase in mortality related to vertebral fracture, although the extent to which this may be due to comorbidities is unclear.

Risk factors for osteoporosis

Non-modifiable

- Increasing age
- Female gender
- Caucasian and Asian population
- Positive family history
- Early menopause
- Previous osteoporotic fractures.

Modifiable

- Smoking
- ≥4 units of alcohol per day
- Diet lacking in calcium-rich food
- Physical inactivity
- Low body mass index (BMI).

Secondary osteoporosis

Endocrine
- Type 1 diabetes
- Hyperthyroidism
- Hyperparathyroidism
- Cushing's disease or syndrome
- Male hypogonadism
- Acromegaly
- Hypopituitarism.

Medical
- Chronic liver disease
- Chronic kidney disease
- Inflammatory bowel disease
- Scurvy
- Vitamin D deficiency
- Eating disorders
- Coeliac and Crohn's disease
- Rheumatoid arthritis
- Amyloidosis
- Stroke or other conditions causing prolonged immobility.

Iatrogenic
- Prolonged steroid use
- Chronic heparin therapy
- Certain anti-epileptics (e.g. phenytoin)
- Post hysterectomy, oophorectomy, or gastrectomy
- Chemotherapy (e.g. methotrexate)
- Aluminum-containing antacids.

Physiological
- Pregnancy
- Lactation.

Inherited
- Down's syndrome
- Turner's syndrome
- Marfan's syndrome
- Ehlers–Danlos syndrome
- Homocystinuria
- Osteogenesis imperfecta.

Haematological
- Sickle cell disease
- Leukaemia.

Vertebral compression fracture

A vertebral compression fracture is defined as a reduction in vertebral body height of at least 20% or 4mm. It has a lifetime risk of 16% for women and 5% for men. About 84% of vertebral compression fractures are associated with pain which typically lasts for 4–6 weeks. In addition to pain, deformity, and reduced mobility, vertebral compression fractures can also indirectly lead to many other problems (e.g. deep vein thrombosis and pressure sores because of reduced mobility, urinary retention and infection, eating disorders, weight loss, paralytic ileus, respiratory dysfunction, sleep disturbance, and depression) which often lead to higher mortality. The standard treatment of such fractures used to be bed rest, analgesia, physiotherapy, fall precautions, and spinal bracing supplemented by medications (e.g. hormone replacement therapy, calcium supplements, and bisphosphonates). Some patients fail to benefit from these measures and have severe intractable pain that does not respond to high doses of analgesia. They may require frequent hospitalization with poor quality of life. Besides, bed rest can further aggravate osteoporosis because of accelerated loss of body mass and bone density. The presence of osteoporosis and co-morbid conditions that are common in the elderly population mean that open surgical procedures are rarely undertaken for these fractures. Even when performed, such procedures can fail because of the poor quality of osteoporotic bone.

In recent years vertebroplasty and kyphoplasty have emerged as novel treatments. These techniques involve percutaneous injection of bone cement into the vertebral body with the aim of stabilizing the vertebral fracture, relieving pain, and preventing further loss of vertebral body height. Vertebroplasty was first used by Galibert and colleagues in 1987 for treating painful vertebral angiomas. Kyphoplasty was first used by Mark Reiley, an orthopaedic surgeon. These procedures are generally performed as day-cases unless there are mitigating social circumstances or serious illness requiring inpatient stay. The exact mechanism by which vertebroplasty and kyphoplasty provides pain relief is still unclear. Possible explanations include the following:

- Stabilization of the fracture by cement, which prevents micromotions.
- Thermal effect of injected cement on intra-osseous pain receptors.
- Chemotoxic effect of injected cement on pain receptors.
- Reduction in kyphotic angle (of more relevance in kyphoplasty than in vertebroplasty).
- Restoration of normal spinal anatomy.

Vertebroplasty and kyphoplasty procedures

Indications
- Painful osteoporotic vertebral compression fractures.
- Traumatic non-osteoporotic vertebral compression fractures.
- Pathological compression fractures from metastasis or myeloma.
- Spinal tumors such as chondrosarcoma and haemangiopericytoma.

Contraindications
Absolute
- Uncorrectable coagulopathy
- Active local or systemic infection
- Vertebra plana
- Asymptomatic patient.

Relative
- Presence of neurological symptoms and/or signs
- Lack of surgical back-up.

Assessment
History
- Presenting complaint including nature, site, and radiation of pain
- History of presenting complaint: this is important as the procedure may not relieve pain in long-standing cases
- Past medical and social history to determine the impact of the condition on the patient, especially in activities of daily living and recreation
- Drug history as analgesic requirements may give an indication of pain severity. If patients are on anticoagulants, such as warfarin, they are advised to stop this one week prior to surgery. However, it is not necessary to stop antiplatelet drugs (e.g. aspirin).

Examination
Examination should follow the time-honoured sequence of look, feel, move, and special tests, especially neurological status. Pain from a vertebral fracture usually results in localized tenderness, but in some cases it may be referred distally. Some patients may have intractable back pain without any local tenderness (11% of patients). Even these patients can benefit from the procedure if imaging confirms the acute nature of the vertebral fracture.

Anaesthetic assessment
As the procedure is carried out prone under intravenous sedation and analgesia, all patients should be assessed with regard to their suitability to lie prone for the duration of the surgery (about 15min for each level). If the patient is unable to do this, they should be assessed by the anaesthetist for suitability to undergo general anaesthesia. Most patients who need general anaesthesia for the procedure will require a chest X-ray and ECG as cardiac and respiratory diseases are common in this subset of patients.

In certain cases special tests (e.g. pulmonary function tests and echocardiography) may be needed.

Investigations
Blood tests
- Routine blood test including full blood count, coagulation study, and bone profile.
- Inflammatory markers.

Imaging
- Plain X-ray can provide information about vertebral body height, but further imaging is needed in all cases.
- MRI provides information about the nature of the fracture and the effect on the neural elements. The short tau inversion recovery (STIR) sequence is believed to be indicative of recent symptomatic vertebral fracture, especially when there are multiple compression fractures of doubtful chronology and symptomatology.
- Computed tomography (CT) provides detailed information about bony elements, including pedicle size, and is especially useful if the integrity of the posterior vertebral wall is in question
- Isotope bone scan is very sensitive but non-specific as it is difficult to distinguish uptake due to fracture from that due to degenerative change. It can be negative for up to 2 weeks after a fracture, and can remain positive up to 2 years after a fracture. However, in certain cases of myeloma, the involved vertebrae may not show typical features on MRI; in such cases a bone scan is very useful, particularly when combined with single-photon emission CT (SPECT).

Consent
Informed consent should be obtained prior to the procedure.

Anaesthesia
In most cases titrated intravenous anaesthesia is sufficient. It is supplemented by LA at sites of skin puncture. The procedure can be carried out in the operating theatre or angiogram suite.

Position
The patient lies prone on a radiolucent table, with a patient support frame if required. There should be space for the C-arm fluoroscope to swing from AP to lateral. Biplanar fluoroscopy is useful but may restrict access for the surgeon.

Preparation
It is important that high-quality fluoroscopy is available and the operator is familiar with the requirements of the procedure. The vertebroplasty or kyphoplasty kit of choice and all instruments and cement required should be available. The scrub nurse should be familiar with the kit and the procedure. Once the patient is anaesthetized and positioned, true AP and lateral images are obtained. The vertebral body should be visualized with the two pedicles and the spinous process seen as the eyes and beak of an owl. Sterile preparation and draping are then carried out.

Access

The selected trocar is introduced through one pedicle (unipedicular) for vertebroplasty and through both pedicles (bipedicular) for kyphoplasty. If the pedicle appearance is likened to a clock face, the trocar is introduced in the 10 o'clock position on the left and the 2 o'clock position on the right side. It is introduced with a medial angulation so as not to breach the medial wall but to end up close to the midline in the vertebral body. All advancement of the trocar should be monitored by orthogonal fluoroscopy. Once the trocar is in a satisfactory position, the preparation for cement injection is carried out depending on whether it is a vertebroplasty or a kyphoplasty.

There is no significant difference between the unipedicular and bi-pedicular approaches for vertebroplasty in terms of restoring vertebral body strength, stiffness, and height. Similarly, transpedicular and extra-pedicular approaches for vertebroplasty are equally efficacious in restoring vertebral body strength. The transpedicular technique results in higher stiffness whereas the extrapedicular approach results in greater height restoration; these findings should be borne in mind, especially when deciding the technique of choice in upper thoracic spine. The unipedicular or bipedicular approach for kyphoplasty results in comparable improvement in Oswestry Disability Index (ODI) and VAS pain scores. However, the bipedicular approach results in statistically significant higher height restoration.

In vertebroplasty the inner needle is removed leaving the outer sheath of the trocar in place. The cement is then mixed and introduced via the introducer when it has reached the correct consistency for injection (usually the consistency of toothpaste). This varies between different types of kit and hence it is recommended that the manufacturer's guidelines are followed. The introduction of cement should be done slowly and deliberately under fluoroscopic guidance, keeping a careful lookout for any cement leakage through the vertebrobasilar veins. If any defects have been identified in the vertebral wall, these should be observed carefully and injection stopped if there is any risk of extravasation. Injection is stopped when the vertebral body is adequately filled. The inner needle is placed in the trocar before withdrawal to prevent backflow of cement into the pedicles.

Bipedicular access is used in kyphoplasty. Two trocars are introduced into the vertebral body under fluoroscopic guidance. Once the optimum position has been reached, the inner needles are removed and a handheld drill is used to create a path for the balloons. A tamp is used to clear any debris from the path. The balloons are then introduced into the prepared path in the vertebral body. The balloons are attached to a syringe with a pressure display which has been prefilled with contrast material. The balloons are inflated with the contrast under fluoroscopy control to effect some restoration of height and create a cavity for the bone cement. The manufacturers recommend maximum volumes and pressures and these should be adhered to very strictly to avoid rupturing the balloon and releasing the contrast into the vertebral body, making monitoring of cement injection difficult. Once the balloons have been inflated satisfactorily, the cement is mixed and the volume to be injected is read from the syringe with contrast corresponding to the amount of contrast that was used to inflate the balloons. The balloons are then sequentially deflated and withdrawn. Cement is then injected into the void/cavity created by the balloons under careful fluoroscopic monitoring.

Once cement injection is complete, the needles are introduced into the trocar to withdraw them without allowing back-flow of cement. (Fig. 8.1). If the vertebra re-collapses after deflation of the balloons and prior to cement injection, the two balloons are re-inflated to the previous volume and pressure settings and then one balloon is deflated and removed while keeping the other inflated. Cement is then introduced into the vertebral body from the side that does not contain the inflated balloon.

The skin puncture site is chosen lateral to the pedicle so that when the converging needles reach the entry point for the pedicles they will be at the upper lateral quadrant of the pedicle (Fig. 8.1).

The skin incision is approximately 5mm long to allow the trocar to be passed. The trocar is advanced until bone is felt and fluoroscopy is used to verify the correct approach to the pedicle (Figs. 8.2 and 8.3). In vertebroplasty one trocar is used and aimed to reach as close to the midline of the vertebral body as possible (Fig. 8.2). In kyphoplasty, a bipedicular approach with two trocars is carried out.

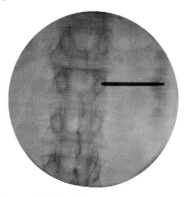

Fig. 8.1 Needle entry to the L1 vertebra.

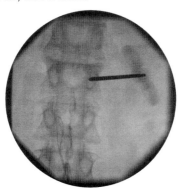

Fig. 8.2 Trocar in the pedicle with intact medial wall.

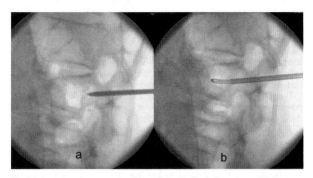

Fig. 8.3 Insertion of trocar and orthogonal images. Once the trocar strikes bone, orthogonal imaging is required to ensure that it follows the optimum path. On AP the medial wall of the pedicle should only be crossed when the tip of the trocar is seen to go past the pedicle and into the vertebral body on lateral views. If the medial wall is breached before this, there is risk of neurological injury (Fig. 8.2).

The next step is drilling and tamping for the balloon path. This step is not required for a vertebroplasty. For kyphoplasty a path needs to be created for the balloons and this is done with a hand-held drill that is introduced into the vertebral body past the outer sleeve of the trocar. This part of the procedure should be done with fluoroscopy to avoid breaching the anterior vertebral wall. Once the path is drilled, a tamp is used to clear bone debris from the drill path. This is an important step to reduce the risk of sharp bone fragments tearing the balloons.

Fig. 8.4(a) shows the balloons being introduced and their position checked. The deflated balloons connected to the contrast syringe are introduced into the path created in the vertebral body and the position is confirmed by fluoroscopy. Fig. 8.4(b)–(d) shows balloons inflated with contrast and the pressure and position checked.

Fig. 8.5 shows the final radiographic result at the completion of vertebroplasty.

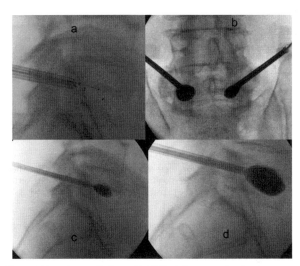

Fig. 8.4 (a) Introduction of balloons. (b)–(d) The balloons are inflated with contrast under fluoroscopic guidance. It is important to inflate slowly and steadily. The syringe is supplied with a pressure monitor and the volume of contrast used can be read from the syringe. Fluoroscopy is used to check that the balloons are sited optimally during inflation. The final volume of contrast used to achieve balloon dilation is noted as this is the volume of cement that will be used. When optimum correction of vertebral height is achieved or when the pressure reaches maximum advisable levels the balloons are sequentially deflated and withdrawn. The cement is supplied in tubes of volume 1.5mL and it is injected under fluoroscopic guidance to ensure that there is no leakage. Once the predetermined volume of cement is injected, the trocar is withdrawn with the stylette inserted to avoid backflow into the pedicles.

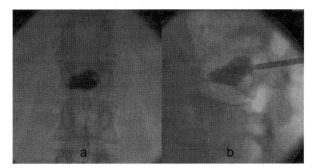

Fig. 8.5 Final radiographic result at completion of vertebroplasty.

Postoperative care

Patients should be monitored with frequent recording of vital signs and neurological status in a designated postoperative observation area on a ward. As the cement normally sets within 20min, there are no restrictions from a mechanical point of view. Usual postoperative nursing care for day-case surgery, including wound check, should be performed, and patients can mobilize when the effects of sedation/anaesthetic have worn off. Once patients have eaten and drunk, passed urine, and are pain free or have pain well controlled with analgesia, they can be discharged home, usually on the day of surgery. Routine follow-up is at 6 weeks, 3 months, and 6 months after the procedure.

Complications

The complication rates for these procedures vary from <2% when treating osteoporotic compression fracture to 10% when treating vertebral compression fracture due to malignancy and include the following:

- Failure of pain relief (5–22%).
- Cement leakage causing increased pain, and weakness or paralysis of limbs including loss of bladder or bowel function (may need emergency surgery). Cement leakage is less common in kyphoplasty (8%) than in vertebroplasty (40%) (3.9% and 2.2% are symptomatic, respectively), as in kyphoplasty, the cement is injected into a low-pressure cavity created by the balloon and the cement is usually of thicker consistency. Recent trials with high-viscosity cement in vertebroplasty have shown cement leakage rates comparable with that of kyphoplasty.
- Infection.
- Haematoma: subdural, epidural, or at puncture site
- Cement or fat embolism: the incidence of pulmonary cement embolus during vertebroplasty and kyphoplasty ranges from 3.5% to 23%, of which the majority is asymptomatic. In general, asymptomatic patients with peripheral pulmonary cement embolus do not require any treatment. Patients with symptomatic and central embolus require treatment in line with the guidelines for management of thromboembolic pulmonary embolism. In rare instances surgical embolectomy (large central pulmonary embolus) or open cardiac surgery (perforation of right ventricle by cement embolus) has been performed.
- Fracture of pedicle, vertebra, or ribs during the procedure.
- Injury to viscera or vessels.
- Stroke.
- Rare complications, e.g. non-aneurysmal subarachnoid haemorrhage, anaphylaxis, lumbar disc herniation, and anterior spinal artery syndrome.
- Patients should be informed that some studies have shown that there may be an increased risk of new vertebral fractures occurring soon after the procedure.

Prognostic factors for the outcome of vertebroplasty in osteoporotic fractures

Better pain relief is seen the following subsets of patients:
- ASA Grade 1
- signal change on the MRI at the treated level
- vertebral body height loss less than 70%
- lower mean T-score
- severe focal back pain
- high-uptake bone scan.

Redo vertebroplasty

Vertebroplasty/kyphoplasty may fail for the following reasons.
- Postoperative infection.
- Use of inadequate cement.
- Adjacent level fracture (8–52% for vertebroplasty and 3–29% for kyphoplasty). Prophylactic vertebroplasty of vertebrae adjacent to fractured vertebrae is controversial.
- Worsening fracture of the treated level.
- Incorrect diagnosis pre-procedure.
- Avascular necrosis of previously treated vertebral body (Kummell's disease). This appears as low signal intensity on T_1 and high signal intensity on T_2 MRI scanning done postoperatively, which is suggestive of fluid collection.

In patients with persistent pain post-procedure, redo vertebroplasty can be performed in certain cases with excellent results, but in other cases anterior or posterior fusion has to be performed.

Routine biopsy during percutaneous vertebroplasty

Routine biopsy should be considered in all patients undergoing percutaneous vertebroplasty for the first time for presumed osteoporotic vertebral compression fracture as it can pick up unsuspected malignancy in 2–3.8% cases. It involves only a marginal increase in operating time and cost, and does not result in increased morbidity or mortality.

Radiation exposure during vertebroplasty

Biplanar fluoroscopy used during the procedure for introduction of the trocar into the vertebral body and to monitor cement filling can lead to significant radiation exposure to the patient (maximum skin dose 0.184–1.834Gy in the AP plane and 0.417–2.362Gy in the lateral plane) as well as to healthcare personnel. All staff must wear appropriate protection to minimize radiation exposure.

Vertebroplasty versus kyphoplasty

A number of studies have compared complications and outcomes of vertebroplasty and kyphoplasty. Controversy still exists about the superiority of one procedure over another. In general they provide comparable pain relief and improvement in VAS/ODI scores. Kyphoplasty results in higher initial restoration of vertebral body height and reduction of kyphotic angle. Vertebroplasty is associated with an increased incidence of cement leak, adjacent level fracture, and symptomatic pulmonary cement embolism. Kyphoplasty is costlier and associated with increased operating time.

Relationship between cement volume, outcome and complications

The amount of cement injected does not correlate with the strength of augmented vertebrae and pain relief. With increased volume of cement used, there is an increase in the risk of cement leak and adjacent level fracture. These phenomena may be interconnected as adjacent level fractures are more common in patients with cement leakage into the disc space than those without a leak (because of the increase in intradiscal pressure and stiffness of the disc). The degree of height restoration with kyphoplasty does not correlate with pain relief.

Important trials in vertebroplasty and kyphoplasty

Efficacy and safety of balloon kyphoplasty compared with non-surgical care for vertebral compression fracture (FREE trial)

- Randomized controlled trial.
- 149 patients assigned to kyphoplasty and 151 assigned to non-surgical care.
- Mean SF-36 physical component summary at 1 month improved from 26 to 33.4 in the kyphoplasty group and from 25.5 to 27.4 in the non-surgical group ($p < 0.0001$).
- Kyphoplasty resulted in greater improvement in quality of life, back pain, and percentage of people requiring opioids compared with the non-surgical group.
- The incidence of adverse events, including new vertebral compression fracture, was the same in both groups.

Percutaneous vertebroplasty compared with optimal pain medication treatment—short-term clinical outcome of patients with subacute or chronic painful osteoporotic vertebral compression fractures (VERTOS study)

- Randomized study.
- 18 patients assigned to vertebroplasty and 16 patients to optimal pain medication.
- Percutaneous vertebroplasty resulted in significantly better VAS scores and less analgesic use 1 day after treatment.
- Two weeks after treatment patients in the vertebroplasty group used significantly less analgesic; they had a better quality of life and improved Roland–Morris Disability Questionnaire scores.
- After 2 weeks, 14 patients managed with optimal pain medication requested vertebroplasty.

Vertebroplasty versus conservative treatment in acute osteoporotic vertebral compression fractures (VERTOS II trial)
- Randomized controlled trial.
- 101 patients assigned to vertebroplasty and 101 assigned to conservative treatment and followed up for 1 year.
- During the study 10% of patients assigned to conservative treatment crossed over to vertebroplasty.
- Difference in mean VAS score between baseline and 1 month was −5.2 for vertebroplasty and −2.7 for controls. Difference in VAS score between baseline and 1 year was −5.7 post-vertebroplasty and −3.7 for controls. The difference was statistically significant at 1 month and 1 year.
- The incidences of cement leak and pulmonary cement embolus after 1 year of follow-up were 72% and 1% respectively. All these patients were asymptomatic.
- During follow-up for new fractures 18 were reported in the vertebroplasty group and 30 in controls. There was no increased vertebral compression fracture post-vertebroplasty.
- Vertebroplasty resulted in a greater improvement in quality of life and decreased analgesia requirements.

Local anaesthesia with bupivacaine and lidocaine for vertebral fracture trial (LABEL trial)
- Unblinded study.
- 19 patients underwent injection of bupivacaine and lidocaine at the site of painful osteoporotic vertebral compression fracture.
- There was no improvement in Roland–Morris Disability Questionnaire scores at rest and average 24h pain at days 1 and 3.
- Pain on activity improved significantly at days 1 and 3.

Controversy surrounding vertebroplasty

In 2009, two studies were published in *The New England Journal of Medicine* which concluded that vertebroplasty was no better than a sham injection of local anaesthetic without cement. Buchbinder and colleagues performed a multicentre randomized double-blind placebo-controlled trial in which 78 patients with one or two painful osteoporotic fractures of less than 12 months duration were assigned to either vertebroplasty or a sham injection. 71 patients completed 6 months follow-up (35 in the vertebroplasty group and 36 in the sham group); outcomes were assessed at 1 week and 1, 3, and 6 months. The study showed that vertebroplasty had no beneficial effect compared with the sham procedure in patients with painful osteoporotic vertebral fractures at any time point. Kallmes and colleagues performed a multicentre randomized trial (INVEST trial) which involved 131 patients with one to three painful osteoporotic vertebral compression fractures who were assigned to either vertebroplasty or a sham injection. The study showed that with regard to pain and pain-related disability in patients with osteoporotic vertebral compression fracture, vertebroplasty had no beneficial effect compared with the sham procedure.

However, there are a number of criticisms of these two studies:
- In both studies, the LA bupivacaine was used in the sham group and may have helped in relieving pain. Though a later trial (LABEL) failed to show similar pain relief with LA injection

- There may also have been selection bias. Buchbinder's group screened 468 patients of which 30% declined to participate and 53% did not meet the eligibility criteria. Similarly, Kallmes' group screened 1813 patients, of whom 16.5% declined to participate and 1382 did not meet the eligibility criteria. Kallmes' group liberalized their inclusion criteria after the start of the trial and 43% of the patients in the sham group had crossed over by 3 months
- The average amount of cement used by Buchbinder's group was 2.8 ± 1.2mL per vertebra. Studies have shown that the smallest amount of cement needed for adequate restoration of vertebral strength is 13–16% of vertebral body volume, i.e. ~4mL of cement at the most commonly treated level at the thoracolumbar junction. Hence a number of patients in the vertebroplasty arm of Buchbinder's study may have had suboptimal treatment
- Vertebroplasty is most effective in patients who have had symptoms for <6 weeks. In the study by Buchbinder's group only 32% of the patients had had symptoms for <6 weeks, and in the study by Kallmes' group the average duration of back pain was 18 weeks
- Inpatients were excluded from the study by Kallmes' group. In general, this subset is most likely to benefit from the procedure.
- The only imaging requirement was plain radiography with MRI being optional; this is not ideal for detecting acute fractures.

Further reading

Breaking point report on osteoporosis (℘ http://www.breakingpoint.org)

Brinjikji W, Comstock BA, Gray L, *et al.* (2010) Local Anesthesia with Bupivacaine and Lidocaine for Vertebral Fracture trial (LABEL): a report of outcomes and comparison with the Investigational Vertebroplasty Efficacy and Safety Trial (INVEST). *AJNR Am J Neuroradiol.* **31**(9):1631–4.

Buchbinder R, Osborne RH, Ebeling PR, *et al.* (2009) A randomized trial of vertebroplasty for painful osteoporotic vertebral fractures. *N Eng J Med* **361**:557–68.

D'Ercole L, Azzaretti A, Thyrion FZ, *et al.* (2010) Measurement of patient skin dose in vertebroplasty using radiochromic dosimetry film. *Spine* **35**(13):1304–6.

Kallmes DF, Comstock BA, Heagerty PJ, *et al.* (2009) A randomized trial of vertebroplasty for osteoporotic spinal fractures. *N Eng J Med* **361**:569–79.

Klazen CA, Lohle PN, de Vries J, *et al.* (2010) Vertebroplasty versus conservative treatment in acute osteoporotic vertebral compression fractures (Vertos II): an open-label randomised trial. *Lancet* **376**(9746):1085–92.

Lee MJ, Dumonski M, Cahill P, *et al.* (2009) Percutaneous treatment of vertebral compression fractures: a meta-analysis of complications. *Spine* **34**(11):1228–32.

McCall T, Cole C, Dailey A (2008) Vertebroplasty and kyphoplasty: a comparative review of efficacy and adverse events. *Curr Rev Musculoskelet Med* **1**(1):17–23.

Muijs SP, Akkermans PA, van Erkel AR, *et al.* (2009) The value of routinely performing a bone biopsy during percutaneous vertebroplasty in treatment of osteoporotic vertebral compression fractures. *Spine* **34**(22):2395–9.

National Institute for Health and Clinical Excellence guidelines on osteoporosis.

Taylor RS, Taylor RJ, Fritzell P (2006) Balloon kyphoplasty and vertebroplasty for vertebral compression fractures: a comparative systematic review of efficacy and safety. *Spine* **31**(23):2747–55.

Voormolen MH, Mali WP, Lohle PN *et al.* (2007) Percutaneous vertebroplasty compared with optimal pain medication treatment: short-term clinical outcome of patients with subacute or chronic painful osteoporotic vertebral compression fractures. The VERTOS study. *AJNR Am J Neuroradiol* **28**(3):555–60.

Wardlaw D, Cummings SR, Van Meirhaeghe J, *et al.* (2009) Efficacy and safety of balloon kyphoplasty compared with non-surgical care for vertebral compression fracture (FREE): a randomised controlled trial. *Lancet* **373**:1016–24.

Spinal cord stimulation in the treatment of chronic pain

S. Eldabe and A. Gulve

Spinal cord stimulation

Introduction

In 1965 the gate control theory revolutionized understanding of chronic pain syndromes. In 1967 it was suggested that stimulating the dorsal columns of the spinal cord would in effect 'close the gate' and control intractable pain in the lower extremities. Since then spinal cord stimulation (SCS) has undergone a variety of technical modifications and has been applied to a variety of pain conditions.

SCS is an effective neuromodulation technique for managing a variety of chronic pain conditions, particularly neuropathic pain that is often refractory to conservative pharmacological and interventional pain management. SCS has also been used to treat ischaemic pain due to peripheral vascular disease, vasospastic conditions, refractory angina pectoris, and intractable visceral pain.

NICE has recommended SCS as a treatment option for adults with chronic pain of neuropathic origin who continue to experience chronic pain (measuring at least 50mm on a 0–100mm VAS) for at least 6 months despite appropriate conventional medical management, and who have had a successful trial of stimulation as part of the assessment.

Indications

Since 1967 SCS has been used to treat many pain problems with variable success. Robust evidence of its benefits in the management of chronic pain has only emerged in the last decade. A number of trials have shown SCS to be an effective technique in the management of pain of neuropathic and vascular or ischaemic origin.

Vascular or ischaemic pain

Refractory angina pectoris

Refractory angina (RA) is defined as a chronic condition characterized by the presence of angina caused by coronary insufficiency in the presence of coronary artery disease that cannot be controlled by a combination of medical therapy, angioplasty, and coronary bypass surgery. The presence of reversible myocardial ischaemia should be clinically established to be the cause of the symptoms. 'Chronic' is defined as duration of more than 3 months. Although the main mechanism of action of SCS in this condition remains unclear, SCS has been shown to reduce pain perception, myocardial oxygen consumption, and sympathetic outflow. It also causes antidromic vasodilatation. There is also evidence for a direct anti-ischaemic effect on the myocardium and improvement in exercise tolerance and electrocardiographic and echocardiographic changes.

The technique for stimulation involves accessing the epidural space via a percutaneous puncture at mid or low thoracic level according to operator preference. An electrode is advanced cranially through the epidural needle so that the tip is lying in the dorsal epidural space at the level of T1 just to the left of the midline. The screening stimulation is then switched on and the settings adjusted to give the patient a sensation of comfortable paraesthesiae over the precordial area and down the left arm as well as in the interscapular region. The electrode is accessed through an incision over the needle and anchored to the surrounding tissue. The electrode is then connected to an implanted pulse generator (IPG) either directly or using an extension cable. The IPG is usually placed in a pocket created in the subcutaneous tissues of the anterior abdominal wall or the buttock area. The patients are advised to switch the stimulator on in response to an attack of angina as well as for prophylaxis before starting any activity that could trigger an angina attack.

Peripheral vascular disease

Patients suffering from peripheral vascular disease (PVD) complain of severe lower-limb pain. The pain is usually worse on movement and amputations are often carried out for pain relief. SCS has been used successfully in the management of PVD pain, particularly in conditions associated with vasospasm such as Raynaud's disease and Buerger's syndrome. SCS is more commonly used in Europe than in the USA.

The technique is similar to that employed in stimulation for RA except that the final electrode tip position in the epidural space is opposite the 9th or 10th thoracic vertebra in the midline to provide paraesthesiae sensations covering both feet and legs and possibly the thighs and buttocks if required. One or two electrodes may be needed to provide complete coverage of the painful area. Screening of SCS is usually conducted to test the efficacy of the therapy before committing to a final implant. The trial involves introducing the electrodes into the epidural space and attaching them to temporary extension(s) to allow time for the patient to experience the sensation and report on the extent of pain relief and paraesthesia coverage. However, there is no clear evidence that screening trials can predict the long-term outcome of SCS in any indication. They are widely practised and generally recommended, but are by no means mandatory.

A number of systematic reviews have shown SCS to be an effective treatment in the management of pain and prevention of amputation in PVD. Patient selection criteria based on a baseline transcutaneous oxygen pressure ($TcPO_2$) ≥20mmHg and an ulcer size <3cm^2 appear to be the most important prognostic factors. Patients who have $>20\%$ increase in $TcPO_2$ during a 2-week trial have better pain reduction as well as limb salvage. PVD sufferers usually use the SCS device at high voltage settings and for prolonged durations during the day and night. This leads to the need for frequent IPG changes. Surgical or plate electrodes have been used to limit the current requirements in this group. These are implanted by a neurosurgeon using an open laminotomy approach to advance a paddle-shaped electrode beneath the laminar arch and place it directly over the dura. Plate or surgical paddle electrodes are generally more stable and lie nearer the dura than percutaneous cylindrical electrodes. The procedure for implanting a surgical electrode is more invasive and has resulted in more procedure-related morbidity. The recent introduction of rechargeable SCS devices has provided an easier solution to the problem of high costs and potential morbidity from frequent surgery for IPG replacement.

Neuropathic pain

Failed back surgery syndrome (FBSS)

FBSS is the most common indication for SCS. FBSS is poorly understood; patients who have undergone anatomically good lumbar or cervical spinal surgery continue to complain of severe spine and limb pain 6 months after surgery. The lumbar syndrome is more common.

Patients with FBSS present with a range of pain distributions, e.g. pain over the lower lumbar spine only or pain over both the lumbar spine and in a radicular distribution in the legs. The limb pain may be unilateral or bilateral.

The technique for SCS involves inserting one or two electrodes with the tip in the lower thoracic spine at the level of T8–10. This usually produces stimulation over both legs and sometimes over the lumbar spine. Axial stimulation is especially difficult to obtain because of the small representation of the lumbar area in the dorsal column fibres of the spinal cord as well as the lateral position of the back fibres around the T9 level, sometimes described as the 'sweet spot'. The need for axial stimulation usually results in high voltage requirements to stimulate back fibres effectively through a thick column of CSF. The high current requirement often results in preferential stimulation of dorsal root fibres, resulting in painful stimulation of the lower thoracic and abdominal wall rather than lumbar stimulation. The use of bipolar electrode configuration has been advocated to focus stimulation on the dorsal column rather than on dorsal root fibres.

Complex regional pain syndrome (CRPS)

Numerous publications describe the value of SCS in reversing the colour, temperature, and pain changes resulting from CRPS. SCS has been used successfully in the management of upper- and lower-limb CRPS types I and II. In upper-limb CRPS the SCS electrode is inserted via an epidural puncture or a laminotomy approach (for a surgical or paddle electrode). The electrode is placed dorsal to the cervical spinal dura between the C4/5 disc cranially and the C8/T1 disc caudally. Some variations on the technique have been described with dual electrodes used to sustain and improve stimulation of the upper limb. Both an anterograde approach, with the electrode inserted from the upper lumbar lower thoracic spine and the tip advanced to rest between T9 and T11, and a retrograde approach, with the electrode inserted via an upper lumbar epidural and advanced in a caudal direction to the L4/5 exit foramen to allow stimulation of the L4, L5, and S1 roots using one electrode, have been described for lower-limb stimulation. Retrograde approach is useful if pain is in the distribution of one or two dermatomes. For non-dermatomal distribution neuropathic pain anterograde approach is recommended.

SCS hardware and technique

Hardware

The main equipment comprises leads (electrode array) and implantable pulse generators which provide power to the electrodes. The electrodes may be unipolar, bipolar, or multipolar, and multiple electrodes may be used. An extension is sometimes used to connect the lead to the pulse generator.

The leads are classified depending on the mode of insertion as percutaneous (cylindrical) or surgical (paddle) leads, and are available in various lengths. Percutaneous leads are subclassified depending on the number of electrodes as quads (four electrodes) and octads (eight electrodes). The inter-electrode distance is also variable. Surgical leads are also called 'paddle electrodes'. They are thicker than percutaneous leads and hence may require a lower amplitude. Surgical leads are available in variety of electrode configurations. All the leads are available in various lengths. The pulse generators can be rechargeable or non-rechargeable systems.

Further details of the hardware can be obtained from the individual manufacturers.

Technique

Trial of SCS

A trial is performed to establish whether the paraesthesiae are covering most of the painful area and are providing acceptable pain relief. It is common practice to connect the electrodes temporarily to an external stimulating device before proceeding to insertion of the IPG. In some centres this trial is performed on the table to confirm that paraesthesiae are covering most of the areas of pain and IPG implantation follows immediately.

Our practice is to suture the leads in a permanent position and connect them to a temporary extension, which is then tunnelled away from the lead insertion site towards the intended IPG implant site. The trial is then run in the patient's own home/workplace over 2–3 weeks. This allows the patient to undergo a period of trial stimulation during which pain relief, functional improvement, and reduction in medication can be assessed. If the outcome of the trial is favourable, the patient may wish to proceed to IPG insertion. In those circumstances the extension wire is cut and the exit wound is allowed to heal. We then proceed with the IPG implant 3–4 weeks later. At the time of the final implant we locate the connector and remove the remaining portion of the extension. A new extension (if required) or the lead is then connected to a pulse generator. This approach increases the likelihood of a positive outcome and reduces failures over the longer term. However, it involves an extra procedure, takes longer, and still has some false positives.

Although a period of trial stimulation has considerable intuitive appeal, its predictive value is uncertain, and it is well-accepted practice to insert electrodes without trial stimulation.

Antibiotics

According to local guidelines.

Percutaneous lead placement

Percutaneous leads are inserted under local or spinal anaesthesia with minimal sedation to facilitate testing of paraesthesiae. This allows intra-operative verification of stimulation projection and hence more accurate placement. However, percutaneous leads are more prone to migration than surgical electrodes.

Anterograde approach to the dorsal epidural space

The patient should be comfortably positioned in the prone position with wedge under the abdomen to offset the natural lumbar lordosis. Fluoroscopic guidance is essential.

A paramedian approach is used. The epidural space is entered at L2/3, L3/4, or L1/2. In order to facilitate easy lead steering in the epidural space a shallow angle of needle insertion is essential. We normally square up the endplate of the vertebra at the intended epidural entry level and mark a radiological midline. The paramedian needle insertion point is then selected two vertebral levels below at the medial pedicular line. Under continuous fluoroscopy, with the loss of resistance to air technique, a Tuohy needle is passed towards the intended radiological midline in an anterograde direction.

Entry to the epidural space is confirmed by inserting a guidewire until it just comes out of the tip of the needle. The percutaneous lead is then inserted in the desired location. If required, another lead can be placed parallel to the initial lead from the opposite side or the same side.

Once the leads are in a satisfactory anatomical location, intraoperative testing should be carried out to ensure that the paraesthesiae produced are covering the painful areas. Once the patient feels paraesthesia in the desired location, the needles should be removed under continuous fluoroscopy, taking care not to disturb the lead position. The leads are then secured to the supraspinous ligament with a suitable anchor. If required, an extension is connected and tunnelled away from the incision site to the site of the IPG.

Retrograde cephalocaudal approach to lumbosacral nerve roots

This approach is useful for sacral nerve stimulation or in patients with well-defined neuropathic pain in the region of one or two nerve roots.

The patient should be comfortably positioned in the prone position with wedge under the abdomen to offset the natural lumbar lordosis. Fluoroscopic guidance is essential. Using the paramedian approach as described earlier, the epidural space is entered at L2/3, L3/4, or L1/2 with retrograde direction of the Tuohy tip needle. As with the anterograde approach, it is important to keep the tip of the needle as close to the radiological midline as possible. The lead is passed under continuous fluoroscopy guidance in the radiological midline until it passes the L5/S1 junction. At this point it is turned towards the desired sacral foramina. If bilateral coverage is required, a second lead can be introduced from the opposite side in a similar manner. Some physicians also use a third mid-line lead, usually an octad lead positioned in the radiological midline of the sacral canal. Once the leads are in a satisfactory anatomical location, intraoperative testing should be carried out to ensure that the paraesthesiae produced cover the painful areas. Once the patient feels paraesthesiae in the desired location, the needles should be removed under continuous fluoroscopy, taking care not to disturb the lead position. The leads are then secured to the supraspinous ligament with a suitable anchor. If required, an extension is connected which is tunnelled away from the incision site to the site of the IPG.

This approach may be difficult in patients who have had previous lower lumbar spine instrumentation or in patients with spondylolisthesis, scar-sensitive dura, or steep lumbosacral angulation. In addition, the learning curve for this technique is quite steep.

Surgical lead placement

Surgical electrodes have a larger contact area, lower battery use, and better geometry and control of stimulation. They are more stable and hence less liable to migrate. However, a small laminotomy is required to introduce the paddle electrode array. This can be performed either under local anaesthesia or spinal anaesthesia, supplemented with conscious sedation, or under general anaesthesia. Procedure under spinal anaesthesia is not possible at higher thoracic and cervical levels. The advantage of local/spinal anaesthesia is that testing for distribution of paraesthesiae can be done on the table and more accurate lead placement can be obtained.

With the patient in the prone position a 3–4cm incision is made in the midline at the desired level for laminotomy (Table 9.1). For lower-extremity coverage this is generally at T10/11 or T11/12. Once the spinous process and lamina are exposed, a small portion of ligamentum flavum and a small piece of lamina are removed (laminotomy) to expose the epidural space. The epidural space is then dilated under fluoroscopic control by a commercial dilator. A dummy lead is then passed in the appropriate position, and finally a permanent surgical lead is placed under fluoroscopy guidance. Once the lead is in a satisfactory anatomical position, intraoperative testing is performed and minor adjustments in lead position are made so that the paraesthesiae cover 80–90% of the painful area. When the lead is correctly placed, it is anchored to the supra-spinous ligament. An extension is then connected to the lead and tunnelled to the desired IPG location. The wound is then closed.

Some centres use somatosensory evoked potential monitoring to guide accurate lead placement under general anaesthesia. There is minimal evidence that this aids placement of SCS leads.

Table 9.1 Surgical lead placement

Location of pain	Lead tip position
Lumbar spine and legs	T8–T11
Feet	T12–L1 (L5/S1 retrograde)
Arms	C3–C5
Heart	T1–T2
Sacral roots	S3 retrograde

IPG implant

The pulse generator should be implanted in the abdomen or the buttocks. Implantation in the superolateral quadrant of the buttock ensures placement in the non-weight bearing area of the buttock. In the abdomen it should be implanted in between the 12th rib and iliac crest. It is essential that the subcutaneous pouch is of adequate depth and size. Adequate haemostasis is essential. If the IPG is implanted too deep, communication with the device and recharging could be difficult. The skin closure should not be under too much tension in order to avoid wound dehiscence. A large pouch will predispose to haematoma/seroma formation or flipping of the generator. Some IPGs have facilities to suture them in the pouch.

Mechanism of action

The biological basis for the effectiveness of SCS is unclear. Its site and mechanism of action differ depending on the level of stimulation in the spinal column. SCS can also affect viscero-somatic reflexes which can modify a variety of physiological functions.

The effects of SCS on different organ systems are listed in Table 9.2. The mechanism of action of SCS may vary depending on the targeted organ. For example, the mode of action for producing pain relief differs significantly when SCS is applied in neuropathic and in ischaemic pain conditions.

Table 9.2 Effects of SCS on target organs

Level of SCS	Target organ	Response to SCS
Cervical	Broncho-alveolar tree	Bronchodilation
	Peripheral blood vessels supplying upper extremities	Peripheral vasodilation
High thoracic	Heart	Stabilization of intrinsic cardiac nervous system
		Reduction of ischaemia and refractory angina pain
		Decreased infarct size
Mid-thoracic	Abdominal viscera	Decreased colonic spasms
		?Improved gut perfusion
Low thoracic	Peripheral blood vessels supplying lower extremities	Peripheral vasodilation
Sacral	Urinary bladder	Decreased bladder spasticity
		Increased volume tolerance

Novel techniques

Sacral nerve stimulation

Sacral nerve stimulation (SNS) is being used for interstitial cystitis (painful bladder syndrome). Mild non-progressive multiple sclerosis, Parkinson's disease, spinal cord injury, paediatric voiding dysfunction, pelvic pain, and faecal incontinence are some other indications for sacral neuro-modulation. SNS should be tried before resorting to the more invasive surgical procedures.

Sacral neuromodulation has been effective in storage (urgency–frequency and urgency incontinence) and emptying (non-obstructive urinary retention) dysfunctions of the bladder. The mechanism of action involved in SNS may be due to either direct activation of efferent fibres to the striated urethral sphincter causing detrusor relaxation or selective activation of afferent fibres causing inhibition at the spinal and supraspinal levels.

In 1997 the Food and Drug Administration (FDA) in the USA approved transforaminal sacral nerve stimulation for urge incontinence, and in 2003 NICE in the UK approved SNS for urge incontinence. Transforaminal SNS using the InterStim system has been successful in patients with idiopathic non-obstructive retention, retention secondary to deafferentation of the bladder after hysterectomy, and Fowler's syndrome.

The traditional anterograde approach to sacral nerve roots in the cauda equina does not produce consistent successful stimulation because of unique anatomical factors. These include a thick dorsal CSF layer, a mobile conus making consistent paraesthesiae very difficult, and the fact that sacral fibres lie deep within the dorsal columns resulting in stimulation of more proximal fibres subserving distal legs, buttocks, and feet.

A cephalocaudal retrograde approach to the sacral nerve roots tends to produce more consistent stimulation at lower amplitudes. The electrodes are stable within the epidural space or sacral root sleeves, the ability to perform symmetrical parallel placement also ensures bilateral coverage, and more than one sacral nerve root can be stimulated with one lead.

Urologists use the sacral transforaminal approach where an electrode is placed through the S3 posterior sacral foramen. Technical failures such as difficulty in locating the S3 foramen, lead migration, and lead fractures are more common with this approach.

Anterograde trans-sacral hiatus is another approach used for SNS. It is technically easier and can be used in patients where a retrograde placement has been difficult because of previous surgeries and spondylolysthesis. However, there is very high risk of infection due to potential contamination of the area. Because of the paucity of subcutaneous tissue, it is difficult to anchor the leads. The incidence of discomfort at the lead insertion site and skin breakdown could be high.

A retrograde laminotomy technique with a paddle electrode array can be used in difficult cases, but requires the expertise of a spinal surgeon.

SCS for gastrointestinal disorders

Functional bowel disorders are a common cause of abdominal cramping, pain, and abnormal bowel habits. There is a strong association between visceral and possibly somatic hypersensitivity in patients with irritable bowel syndrome arising from abnormalities in the complex bidirectional communication between the central nervous system and the enteric nervous system.

Complications of SCS

Worldwide, over 25,000 neurostimulation devices are implanted every year. With this explosion in the use of implants, related complications have been reported. There have been no prospective studies designed specifically to examine the complications of neurostimulation. The reports tend to be observational and anecdotal. Neurostimulation complications can be broadly divided into two groups: biological and hardware-related.

Biological complications

Infection

Infection is a serious complication of any implant surgery. The typical rate of infection for SCS procedures is ~5%. An infection can present at any time, from a few days after implant to several years later. *Staphylococcus aureus* is the most common organism involved in SCS infections. Many studies have shown the IPG pocket site to be the most common location of infection. The treatment is removal of the complete system and treatment with intravenous antibiotics. If the infection is confined to the IPG site, it may be possible to remove the IPG only and treat the patient with antibiotics, leaving the electrodes in place. This is a risky strategy and it may make it more difficult to eliminate the infection. Subsequent electrode removal is often required. Both septic and aseptic meningitis have been reported after SCS. There is a case report of paralysis after epidural and intradural abscess formation at an electrode tip. Despite electrode removal and abscess debridement recovery was incomplete. Infection prevention techniques include administration of prophylactic antibiotics, adequate skin preparation, meticulous attention to sterile techniques in the operating room, and adequate wound haemostasis.

Dural puncture

Accidental dural puncture can occur during epidural needle placement for electrode positioning. This can result in postdural puncture headache symptoms as well as CSF leak into the wound. The incidence of dural puncture is 0–0.3%. Patients who experience postdural puncture headache may suffer from a positional headache, diplopia, tinnitus, neck pain, photophobia, and fluid accumulation at the electrode anchoring site. These patients will be unable to perform activities of daily living and are therefore unable to assess the efficacy of an SCS trial. Blood patching is hazardous in such cases because of infection risk.

Neurological injury

Neurological injury is the most dreaded complication of SCS. It can result from direct trauma caused by epidural needle puncture or percutaneous electrode placement, or occur during surgery for placement of paddle electrodes. Delayed neurological damage can result from epidural haematoma or abscess formation. Epidural haematoma formation following placement of SCS electrodes is rare.

Hardware complications

Hardware complications are far more common in SCS therapy than biological complications. Most only result in minor morbidity and can be remedied with limited surgical revision procedures. However, hardware complication can result in patient dissatisfaction and an increase in the economic burden on the healthcare system. The most common hardware complication is electrode migration, which results in shift of paraesthesiae. Most require a further surgical procedure to revise the position of the electrode, but some can be remedied by reprogramming. X-ray examination of the electrode position is usually diagnostic when compared with the original electrode position films. Despite the high rate of complications, most are minor and often hardware related. The majority require further surgery to restore device effectiveness.

Conclusion

SCS is a minimally invasive and fully reversible non-drug treatment which is effective for a number of pain conditions. It may allow the patient and physician a trial period to assess the effectiveness of the device and the extent of paraesthesiae coverage. Some centres conduct trials of varying duration (a few minutes to a few weeks) and some do not. The last decade has seen the emergence of good evidence of the effectiveness and cost-effectiveness of SCS in FBSS and CRPS. Further evidence, particularly for ischaemic pain, remains an issue. Despite the emerging evidence, the place of SCS in a pain treatment algorithm continues to depend on individual physician perceptions and practices. As yet, no clear guidance can place SCS at a particular step on the treatment continuum.

Pearls of wisdom

- SCS is an effective therapy for treating neuropathic pain.
- For the best outcome SCS paraesthesiae should cover most of the area of pain.
- MRI examination of any part of the body should not be conducted on a patient with an implanted spinal cord stimulator using an RF transmit body coil.

Further reading

Holsheimer J (1998). Computer modelling of spinal cord stimulation and its contribution to therapeutic efficacy. *Spinal Cord* **36**; 531–40.

Kumar K, Taylor RS, Jacques L, *et al.* (2007). Spinal cord stimulation versus conventional medical management for neuropathic pain: a multicentre randomised controlled trial in patients with failed back surgery syndrome. *Pain* **132**:179–88.

Linderoth B, Foreman RD, Meyerson BA (2009). Mechanisms of action of spinal cord stimulation. In Lozano AM, Gildenberg PL, Tasker RR (eds), *Textbook of Stereotactic and Functional Neurosurgery* (2nd edn), pp 2331–47. Berlin: Springer-Verlag.

NICE (2008). *Technology Appraisal—Pain and Spinal Cord Stimulation*. Available online at: http://www.nice.org.uk/guidance/index.jsp?action=byID&o=11739.

North RB, Kidd DH, Farrokhi F, Piantadosi SA (2005). Spinal cord stimulation versus repeated lumbosacral spine surgery for chronic pain: a randomized, controlled trial. *Neurosurgery* **56**:98–107.

Taylor RS, Ryan J, O'Donnell R, Eldabe S, Kumar K, North RB (2010). The cost-effectiveness of spinal cord stimulation in the treatment of failed back surgery syndrome. *Clin J Pain* **26**:463–9.

Intrathecal drug delivery

L. Lynch

Intrathecal drug delivery

Introduction

Intrathecal drug delivery (ITDD) has been an option for the management of persistent pain since the 1980s. The discovery of opioid receptors in the central nervous system in 1976 was the impetus for early attempts to deliver opioids intraspinally.

ITDD is currently used in the management of patients with both cancer-related pain and severe intractable nociceptive and neuropathic pain of other origins and in the management of spasticity.

In this chapter we consider some of the practical aspects of the rationale behind the treatment, patient selection, drugs, available systems and implant technique, aftercare and complications, and potential future developments.

Systems used to deliver intrathecal (IT) drugs can either utilize a fully implanted programmable or fixed-rate infusion pump or a tunnelled catheter or port access leading to an external pump. In this chapter we will only consider the fully implanted systems, although we will make reference to external systems in the management of the late stages of cancer-related pain.

Background

The advantage of ITDD is that in selected patients it has the promise of improved efficacy and reduced side effects compared with other routes of drug administration. Improvements in function, quality of life, and even life expectancy for cancer patients come as part of the package.

The disadvantages and problems of ITDD are significant and limit the use of systems in patients without cancer-related pain.

Relevant spinal anatomy and CSF fluid dynamics

It is important to understand the anatomy of the spinal cord and IT space and the characteristics of CSF circulation that affect drug distribution. An understanding of drug pharmacokinetics is also essential to predict how to place IT catheters and how to use the different drugs to deliver adequate doses to the right place in the spinal cord so that the pharmacodynamics is able to work.

The aim of an ITDD system is to deliver the relevant drug to the appropriate site in the dorsal horn at a sufficient dose to be effective. Knowledge of CSF dynamics helps to optimize drug perfusion rates, penetration depths, and targeted drug delivery.

It has become clear that CSF does not flow from its sites of production in the ventricles (and elsewhere) down to the spinal cord and then back again. Instead, the evidence points to CSF circulating around the cord in a series of segmental 'doughnuts' with no overall flow at all. The CSF does not distribute drugs by flowing around the neuraxis as previously believed.

Slow continuous infusions (e.g. 20μL/h) such as those from implanted ITDD systems do not distribute drugs beyond the 'doughnut' adjacent to the catheter port. A slow bolus (maximum rate 1mL/h) from these systems probably only distributes the drug more widely within the bolus. It is worth noting that a single-shot anaesthetic bolus (e.g. 2.5mL over a couple of seconds, often with 'a bit of baboutage') distributes the drug much more widely and breaks through the constraints of local fluid movement.

Therefore it seems intuitive that the catheter tip should be positioned at least at, and possibly above, the dermatomal level of the patient's pain. Similarly, the catheter is best placed posterior to the spinal cord, rather than anterior.

Drug factors (i.e. physicochemical properties and pharmacokinetics) are important and this in part determines the way that the drug is partitioned into the grey matter, white matter, blood, and fat. For example, because of its physicochemical properties and pharmacokinetics, ziconotide is distributed widely in the neuraxis. Therefore catheter position is not as crucial as for a minimally distributed drug like hydromorphone or bupivacaine.

The pharmacokinetics of IT drugs is a function of their lipid solubility. Lipid-soluble opioids are cleared rapidly from CSF to the fat of the epidural space and into the plasma. This means that they are likely to be less well distributed in the CSF than hydrophilic dugs like morphine.

Drug spread in the CSF depends on buoyancy, streaming, injection rate, and enhanced diffusion. Diffusion alone is not helpful—it takes 24 hours for a drug to move 1cm.

Drugs

Only morphine and ziconotide are licensed for ITDD. Only drugs free from preservatives and additives should be used in IT therapy because of the potential neurotoxicty of these chemicals and their potential to interact with CSF proteins and cause catheter blockage.

A consensus group at the World Institute of Pain's International Meeting in New York City in 2007 developed a polyanalgesic algorithm for IT therapies (Table 10.1) based on a review of literature from PubMed, EMBASE, and Google Scholar from 1966 onwards.

Opioids work pre- and postsynaptically by depressing neuro-transmitter release and hyperpolarizing the membranes of neurons in the dorsal horn. The μ-opioid receptor is linked to presynaptic calcium channels via a G-protein-coupled mechanism. Opioids inhibit this channel, but indirectly and partially as not all μ receptors are linked to calcium channels. With time there is a functional uncoupling of the link, reflected clinically by the development of tolerance.

Serious adverse opioid-related effects include opioid-induced hyper-algesia, hypotension, sedation, respiratory depression, and hypogonado-tropic hypogonadism which can result in sexual dysfunction and osteo-porosis. Supraspinal effects are more likely with the less lipophilic drugs; there is more risk of respiratory depression with morphine than with hydromorphone.

Table 10.1 Polyanalgesic algorithm for IT therapies

First line	Morphine or
	Hydromorphone or
	Ziconotide
Second line	Fentanyl or
	Morphine/hydromorphone + ziconotide
	Morphine/hydromorphone + bupivacaine/clonidine
Third line	Clonidine
	Morphine/hydromorphone/fentanyl/bupivacaine + clonidine + ziconotide
Fourth line	Sufentanil
	Sufentanil + bupivacaine + clonidine + ziconotide
Fifth line	Ropivacaine
	Buprenorphine
	Midazolam
	Meperidine
	Ketorolac
Sixth line	Experimental agents: gabapentin, octreotide, conpeptide, neostigmine, adenosine, XEN2174, AM336, XEN, ZGX160

Morphine

Morphine is the most commonly used opioid available and it is approved by the FDA. It is a relatively small hydrophilic molecule (molecular weight 285Da) and is water soluble.

Morphine has a slow onset and a long duration of action relative to other opioids, with a half-life in CSF of 80min, but it has problems with tolerance, hyperalgesia, IT granulomas, and endocrine effects. A conversion factor of 1mg IT morphine equivalent to 300mg oral morphine equivalents is often cited. It can be used in combinations with LAs and clonidine.

Hydromorphone

Hydromorphone is a synthetic opioid which is both more lipophilic and more potent (4–7×) than morphine. Fewer supraspinal effects are reported. It is more stable than morphine with ziconotide. It can be used in combination with clonidine and bupivacaine.

Bupivacaine

Bupivacaine and levobupivacaine (the s-optical isomer of bupivacaine) work by sodium-channel blockade and are effective for both nociceptive and neuropathic pain. Bupivacaine can be used alone or in combination with opioids and clonidine. Tachyphylaxis occurs and the effect of high-dose infusion is only short term. Boluses are a more effective way of using the drug, often at very low doses (2mg or less).

There is certainly evidence in rats that LAs are neurotoxic and there are some reports of neurotoxicity in humans when high concentrations of lidocaine have been used in IT. Neurotoxicity is dose-related in animals and so low concentrations may well be safe. Continous high concentrations of bupivacaine may best be reserved for patients with cancer-related pain.

Fentanyl

Fentanyl is highly lipophilic μ-agonist that is not currently used for longer-term IT infusions, but well used anaesthetically. There is no evidence of granuloma formation, probably as the drug is absorbed very rapidly across the dura compared with either morphine or hydromorphone. There may be potential for use with a patient therapy manager.

Sufentanil

Sufentanil has similar features to fentanyl, but is not available in the UK.

Clonidine

Clonidine is an α_2-adrenoceptor agonist that binds to both pre- and post-synaptic α_2-receptors in the dorsal horn. It acts by reducing the release of C-fibre neurotransmitters, such as substance P and calcitonin-gene-related peptide (CGRP), and possibly by also reducing preganglionic sympathetic outflow. It also causes hyperpolarization of the postsynaptic membrane via a G-coupled potassium channel.

It is effective for neuropathic pain in IT doses of 60–1000micrograms/ day. It has a synergistic antinociceptive interaction with other drugs, no tolerance, and may be protective against granuloma formation. It is the most stable drug in combination with ziconotide. However, abrupt withdrawal can be fatal and any reduction in doses needs to be gradual.

Ziconotide

This is a new class of IT drug (an n-type calcium-channel blocker and non-opioid analgesic) and has only recently become available, so neither the optimum administration strategies nor its role in pain management are established as yet. It has been recommended as the first-line IT agent in the management of chronic pain of all varieties, both nociceptive and neuropathic. There is no evidence of granuloma formation and no evidence of tolerance.

Ziconotide is a synthetic analogue of ω-conotoxin which originates from the fish-eating marine snail *Conus magnus*. The snail uses a mix of conotoxins to kill its prey within seconds. The molecule itself is large, comprising 25 amino acids and weighing 2659Da. It is completely ionized at physiological pH, freely soluble in water, and therefore hydrophilic. Most other IT drugs are small un-ionized molecules.

The exact mechanism of action in humans is unknown, but animal work shows it to be a selective inhibitor of presynaptic n-type calcium channels which are concentrated in the superficial laminae (I and II) of the dorsal horn of the spinal cord. These calcium channels are blocked directly by ziconotide and indirectly by opioids. Tolerance does not develop with ziconotide, unlike opioids.

Ziconotide can only be used intrathecally. It was approved for the treatment of chronic severe pain by the FDA in December 2004 and by the European Medicines Evaluation Agency (EMEA) in February 2005. It is recommended for use in all types of pain—the polyanalgesic consensus of 2007 (Table 10.1) recommended it as a first-line treatment for noci-ceptive, mixed, and neuropathic pain.

Ziconotide is contraindicated in patients on IT chemotherapy and those with a clinically defined psychosis.

Pharmacokinetics

Ziconotide is only suitable for IT administration and is distributed widely throughout the neuraxis, unlike any other agent in use. Radiolabelled ziconotide in rats reaches the neocortex, basal ganglia, forebrain, hippocampus, olfactory glomerulus, and dorsal grey matter, as well as the CSF and superficial dorsal horn.

The volume of distribution in the CSF is the same as the CSF volume (~140mL). The CSF clearance is approximately equal to the CSF turnover rate of 0.3–0.4mL/min.

Ziconotide is not metabolized in the CSF, but when it reaches the systemic circulation it is rapidly metabolized by ubiquitous proteolytic enzymes with 50% being bound in the plasma protein. It has a terminal half-life in CSFof 4.6h an average.

It is present in the systemic circulation in only very low concentrations and so no dose reduction is necessary in patients with either liver or renal impairment. There is virtually no interaction with any other systemic medications.

The maximum drug distribution is reached within 24h but pain relief and side effects take between 2 and 28 days of any dose alteration to manifest. Slow titration regimens are recommended and are discussed in 'Infusion regimens and management post-implant' p.182.

Neurological adverse events are common and are related to the drug distribution in higher centres. The top ten are as follows.

- Neurological:
  - dizziness (53%)
  - headache (35%)
  - nystagmus (30%)
  - somnolence (27%)
  - memory impairment (22%)
  - abnormal gait (21%).
- Gastrointestinal:
  - nausea (51%)
  - vomiting (19%)
  - constipation (19%).
- Whole body:
  - fever (20%).

Most adverse events are reported as mild to moderate and transient. All will stop with cessation of drug infusion, although this may take weeks.

Creatine kinase levels may rise during therapy, and a baseline level should be recorded prior to treatment and at intervals throughout. If there is a progressive rise, there is a risk of myopathy and rhabdo-myolysis and the infusion should be stopped.

Other drugs

Other drugs have been used IT and more are being tested, but none of those discussed here are in regular usage:

Buprenorphine

Buprenorphine is a semi-synthetic opioid derived from thebaine. It is regarded as a partial μ-opioid receptor agonist and a κ- and δ-opioid receptor antagonist, but in clinical practice it behaves as a pure μ-agonist. It is five times as lipid soluble as morphine and 25–30 times as potent. It dissociates very slowly once bound to its receptor and so has a relatively long duration of action and only low levels of receptor occupancy (5–10%) produce analgesia.

Midazolam

Midazolam is available only with preservative which prevents normal usage. It is an imidazobenzodiazepine with unique properties compared with other benzodiazepines. It is highly water soluble at pH <4 and highly lipid soluble at pH >4. Benzodiazepine receptors are allosteric modulatory sites close to GABAa receptors, and benzodiazepines work by enhancing the interaction of GABA (γ-aminobutyric acid) with its receptors by increasing the frequency of chloride ion channel opening. The neuronal membrane is hyperpolarized and less able to depolarize in response to excitatory neurotransmitters—the overall effect is inhibitory. Research indicates analgesia without major adverse effects, but rat studies raise the possibility of neurotoxicity.

Ketorolac

Ketorolac is a water-soluble NSAID which works by inhibiting both cyclo-oxygenase (COX) isoenzymes. The theory is that prostaglandins have a role in hyperalgesia secondary to tissue injury and inflammation. Therefore COX inhibitors can potentially prevent escalation of this cascade of circulating cytokines and sensitization of spinal nociceptive processing.

The doses needed to do this systemically give too many side effects (gastric ulceration, renal blood flow, and platelet inhibition), whereas the doses needed intrathecally are 100–300 times lower.

There does not seem to be any untoward spinal toxicity in rats and dogs, although very high IT doses as chronic continuous infusions can result in systemic side effects. Suppression of prostaglandin levels in the CSF seems to be greater with continuous infusions than with bolus administration.

'Experimental' agents

'Experimental' agents include gabapentin, octreotide, corpeptide, neostigmine, adenosine, XEN2174, AM336, XEN, and ZGX160.

Neostigmine

Neostigmine is a selective reversible acetylcholinesterase inhibitor. Higher levels of acetyl choline enhance analgesia via muscarinic binding sites in the dorsal horn; 50–200micrograms have been used as IT boluses in the management of postoperative and chronic neuropathic pain states. There is no evidence of toxicity, but bradycardia and nausea are frequent side effects.

Gabapentin

Gabapentin is a GABA analogue which probably works by binding to the $\alpha_2\delta$ subunit of a voltage-gated calcium channel and reducing glutamate in the dorsal horn. It may also work by activating noradrenergic mechanisms. The theoretical advantage of using gabapentin intrathecally is that it has a saturable active transport system in both the gut and across the blood–brain barrier.

Octreotide

Octreotide is a synthetic octapeptide analogue of the growth hormone somatostatin which is found in the substantia gelatinosa and is associated with analgesia. Analgesia has been reported in animal and human studies with octreotide doses of 405–650micrograms/day. Tolerance may develop.

Adenosine

Adenosine is an endogenous purine nucleoside which subserves many functions by binding to four types of receptor: A1, A2A, A2B, and A3. The A1 receptors are found in brain and spinal cord, and mediate anti-nociception. There are some A2A receptors on GABA-ergic neurons. All the receptors are G-protein coupled.

Contraindicated drugs

Ketamine
Ketamine, an *N*-methyl-D-aspartate (NMDA) receptor antagonist, causes widespread spinal necrosis with haemorrhage, vaccuolation, and myelin loss, microglial activation, and chromatolysis when infused IT in humans. This has been confirmed in human post-mortem studies and rabbit models.

Methadone
Methadone produces isomer-specific neurotoxicity.

Diamorphine
Diamorphine has been used with great success, but is now contra-indicated following reports of breakdown products causing pump stall.

Patient selection

Theoretically any patient with severe intractable chronic pain originating below the brainstem, unrelieved by best medical management (medication/interventions/supportive therapy) may be a candidate. This includes those with opioid-sensitive pain who are unable to tolerate opioid side effects. There are two distinct groups: those with chronic non-malignant pain (CNMP), and those with cancer-related pain (CP). Ziconotide may have an effect above brainstem level.

It is worth emphasizing that a thorough medical assessment of the patient is mandatory. The treatment of any pain condition is the treatment of its cause, and this needs to be clear. Further investigation and opinions may be needed and may lead to other treatment opportunities, and sometimes to definitive treatment.

Spinal imaging is extremely useful at this stage both to delineate spinal anatomy and as a baseline if further imaging is required in the future. Undiagnosed/impending cord compression can be seen in the pre-operative work-up of the CP patient. MRI is possible with an implanted pump, but may lead to stalling of the rotor arm in fully implanted programmable systems and a period of time without ITDD.

The selection of CNMP patients must be 'by a multiprofessional team with a comprehensive understanding of the physical, psychological, and rehabilitation aspects of the patient's condition' (from the British Psychological Society guidelines for best clinical practice). This is not mandatory for CP patients with a very limited life expectancy, and ITDD may still be indicated even for patients with serious psychological/psychiatric/personality disorders or issues, and each case would have to be considered on its merits. The advice of a liaison psychiatrist or psychologist with experience of patients with cancer and CP can always be sought. The ability to give informed consent and to understand the technique and its implications may be a problem for some. Some CP patients are so sedated pre-implant that psychological issues are just not evident until sedative drugs are reduced.

Catheter position is a limiting factor, with significant adverse drug effects above T4 due to effects on cardiac fibres, although ITDD can be used for refractory angina. For example, the catheter may have to be positioned at C4 or C5 for a patient with recurrent progressive breast cancer and tumour invading the brachial plexus, and the doses of drugs required to be effective may well have prohibitive side effects.

Ideally, catheters should be inserted below the level of the spinal cord and advanced upwards. The higher the catheter position, the more difficult the positioning may be.

Spinal canal deformities and tumours, along with a history of impending or actual cord compression, can present difficulties Previous spinal surgery can present anatomical difficulties with IT catheterization or siting of the catheter at the appropriate level.

Infection is a contraindication because of the risk to the implanted system/catheter of local pump pocket infection and meningitis. However, low-grade infections related to tumours may be manageable with antibiotics. It is worth mentioning that progressive tumours are associated with a progressive rise in CRP. Obviously a site of infection should be sought, but if an infection screen is negative it may well be acceptable to proceed.

Bleeding diatheses are another contraindication. Anticoagulated patients can be managed as per haematology/anaesthetic protocols.

Pre-existing foot and leg oedema and venous insufficiency predispose to ongoing problems, particularly with opioid infusions, and are relative contraindications.

A 3–6-month cut-off for likely survival is often quoted for implants for CP management. This is based on a financial analysis. It is certainly not a technique for the terminal stages of life when external systems or other management would be appropriate, but an apparently almost moribund, heavily sedated, but distressed patient with inadequate pain control may be transformed and live for many months.

The willingness of a patient to travel for necessary refills needs to be established prior to implant unless the treating team is able to offer an 'at-home' service.

Examples of patients with non-cancer pain who may be suitable for IT pumps include (in no particular order):

- spinal pain
- abdominal pain
- haematuria loin pain syndrome
- ischaemic pain
- chronic refractory angina.

Types of ITDD system

Systems can be divided into those using either external or fully implanted pumps.

External pumps must be specific for ITDD. They can be used with either a percutaneous catheter (tunnelled or untunnelled) or a totally implanted catheter with a subcutaneous injection port. All have an increased infection rate compared with the fully implanted system. Highest infection rates occur with untunnelled catheters, followed by tunnelled and then implanted catheters. The advantage of external pumps is that they are easily and quickly sited and relatively cheap in terms of time and equipment needed. However, there is more of a chance of infection and catheter migration, and the pump itself is relatively bulky. They are suitable for use on a trial basis and for patients with a limited life expectancy. Depending on the staff and infrastructure available, patients may have to be managed as inpatients in a hospital or hospice. Trained staff are essential throughout all tiers of patient care. External pumps are particularly effective for end-of-life care, as they can infuse much larger volumes than is possible from the finite reservoirs and limited rates of infusion of the fully implanted systems.

Fully implanted pump systems are either fixed-rate or programmable. The programmable systems may have a bolus facility and the possibility of a patient-controlled bolus facility. These systems are ideal for longer-term use and have a substantially reduced risk of infection. They are more convenient and do not limit patient activity to the same degree as the external pumps. They can be managed entirely at home except for a commitment to return for regular refills. Fully implanted pumps are gas driven, fixed-rate, or battery-powered programmable.

Fixed-rate pumps have the potential to last for the lifespan of the patient as they do not have a limited-life power source. They are cheaper, but it is not possible to change drug infusion regimens without changing the drug concentration or constituents in the reservoir. It is also impossible to turn off the pump—the reservoir must be emptied.

Programmable pumps have the flexibility of dose adjustments with an obligatory refill. They are battery driven with a lifespan of up to 8 years. One of the programmable pumps has a 'patient therapy manager' which allows the patient to administer a preset IT bolus, giving enormous flexibility in pain control, particularly for CP patients.

Currently available pumps

Medtronic

Only the Synchromed II is currently available, but the Isomed and Synchromed EL will still be implanted in some patients.

The Synchromed II is a programmable titanium pump with a reservoir of either 20 or 40mL (model numbers 8637-20 and 8637-40, respectively). It has a diameter of slightly less than 9cm and weighs 165–175g when empty and 185–215g when full. It has a battery-powered motor and electronics that will last for 6–7 years with normal usage. It has a bacterial filter and a silicone central port which is designed for 500 punctures. There is a side access port with direct access to the spinal IT catheter and therefore the CSF. It is possible to access the CSF through this port, either for sampling in possible cases of infection or for direct bolusing of analgesics or antibiotics.

The minimum flow rate is 0.048mL/day and the maximum is 1mL/h. The pump can be programmed to deliver simple continuous infusions or complex variable-rate infusions. The current programming unit is known as the N-vision.

Medtronic are the only manufacturer to offer a patient-controlled bolusing device—the 'patient therapy manager' (PTM). This can be programmed via the pump using the N-vision. The bolus itself is set in units of the primary drug (e.g. 2mg of bupivacaine). The duration of the bolus is set in minutes with the proviso that the pump can deliver a maximum rate of 1mL/h. For example, for 4% bupivacaine (40mg/mL) and a bolus of 2mg, the minimum duration would be 3min. The minimum duration for a bolus of 5mg would be 8min and so on. The duration of infusion of the bolus can be extended if the more rapid infusion rates produce side effects (e.g. dizziness, hypotension, numbness, urinary incontinence). The lockout interval and the maximum number of activations per 24h period can be programmed. Time zero is the time at which the programming episode takes place (not midnight) and the lockout interval is timed from the end of the bolus infusion (not from the start of the last bolus).

The pump has one alarm, a volume alarm, which can be turned off. The volume is calculated from the programming information, i.e. if the programme set to deliver a volume of 40mL at a rate of 1mL/day and the volume alarm is set at 1mL then the pump will alarm after 39 days whatever the actual volume in the pump. If a background rate of 0.5mL/day has been set with a maximum bolus facility of 7 × 0.5mL, the pump will alarm when it calculates that 1mL is left. The alarm date given with the programming information is simple in the first example, but in the second example it is calculated by assuming that the maximum number of potential activations will be used (i.e. 4mL/day), which will give an alarm date after 9 days. If the patient uses one bolus a day on most days and seven during flare-ups, the volume will last much longer.

The major advantage of the PTM is that it allows very flexible dosing regimens which is particularly useful for unstable CP. There is evidence of improved analgesia when bolus-based regimens are used and also of less tolerance and tachyphylaxis developing to opioids and bupivacaine. Use of a low-background infusion with as-required bolusing *may* also reduce granuloma formation. The disadvantage is that bolus-based regimens decrease the time between refills and can substantially reduce battery life.

Codman (Johnson & Johnson)

Codman currently manufacture two types of implantable pump: the Archimedes®, which is a gas-driven constant-flow pump, and the Medstream™, which is a novel programmable variable-rate battery-powered pump. The Archimedes is a circular titanium pump with two access ports—a central refill port and a peripheral catheter access port.

The pump has an inner chamber containing infusate, which leaves through a filter and flow restrictor to the spinal catheter, and an outer chamber containing propellant. The pumps have a constant infusion rate, so in order to change the amount of drug delivered, the concentration of the infusate has to be changed. The pump is available in reservoir volumes of 20, 35, 40, 50, and 60mL and flow rates of 0.5, 0.8, 1.0, 1.3, 1.5, 2.0, and 3.0mL/day. The lifespan of the pump is a reflection of the lifespan of the silicone membrane of the central refill port, and is generally ~10 years. The Medstream pump features a ceramic drive system, which has no motors, gears, or rotating parts, and a lithium–carbon monofluoride battery with an 8 year lifespan independent of flow rate. Two reservoir volumes are available: 20mL or 40mL. The minimum flow rate is 0.004mL/h and the maximum flow rate is 0.167mL/h. There are three alarms: a critical alarm for pump hardware failure and two non-critical alarms, one indicating battery life within 3 months and the other, connected to a fill-level sensor measuring the true volume of infusate, indicating a reservoir volume <3mL.

Patient information sessions

Prior to listing for implant, a relaxed information session with an opportunity to view the equipment and consideration of the implications is invaluable. The pump itself is about the size of a standard tin of tuna; much too large for some to contemplate as an implant but neat and convenient for the majority. The concerns of patients regarding their pumps are not the same as those of their physicians. They have an interest in the mechanics and the medication, but they want to know about limitations and how it will affect everyday life. Deep sea diving is no great loss to most people, but most would still like to fly for holidays and want to know if this is possible—it is.

Test doses and trials

The consensus view of trials and test doses is that some form of trial is generally recommended, but there are no rules as to how this should be conducted and no easily available or simple test kit to use for infusions. Local factors including funding, availability of patient in-patient beds and staffing, have a huge impact on what is feasible.

An ideal trial would need to reproduce the features of the fully implanted system and would probably comprise the implantation of a catheter at the correct level for the patient's pain (or possibly mid-thoracic for ziconotide) attached to a subcutaneous port access system and then to an external pump capable of flow rates similar to the definitive systems (e.g. the CADD MS pump which can deliver flow rates of 20µL/h. However, it could be argued that cancer patients, particularly children and teenagers with terminal cancer, form a different group.

Bolus trials have the advantage of being 'easy' in terms of the equipment needed and the time involved, but they do not replicate the features of any implanted system in current use, even those with a bolus facility. The maximum rate of infusion of a bolus from the Medtronic Synchromed II pump is 1mL/h—not 1mL over 1s! However, they can still be used to predict whether or not the drugs used will be effective. Infusion regimens are described later.

Boluses can be of either a single drug or a combination. Outcomes of ziconotide bolus trials are awaited, but trials of opioids have already been described. LA can be used alone or with an opioid, and clonidine can also be added. Placebos have also been used.

A national survey of practice in Canada revealed that practitioners used boluses of 0.03–3mg morphine with 18–27G spinal needles. The average conversion factor from oral morphine equivalents was 1/300 (1/100–1/600). Boluses were repeated by 73% of responders.

A study of the predictive value of IT opioid trials using three sequential boluses followed by one or two single blinded placebo injections identified three dose ranges for morphine (0.25mg–0.5mg–1.0mg), hydromorphone (0.0625mg–0.125mg–0.25mg), and sufentanil (2.5micrograms–5micrograms–10micrograms).

In our cancer pain practice, we use hydromorphone, clonidine, and bupivacaine. We use a conversion factor for hydromorphone of 1/200 of oral morphine equivalents. For a single bolus we use a 12h dose, ie 1/400 of the 24h oral morphine equivalent dose. For example, we would use a bolus of 2.5mg for a patient having 1000mg/day oral morphine equivalent. Our suggested maximum is 5mg hydromorphone. Clonidine can be added, and we use 15–30micrograms in a bolus (combined with hydromorphone 9 bupivacaine). For mixed pain we add usually 2–5mg bupivacaine. For opioid-sensitive pain we would expect at least 12h (often up to 24–48h) of good analgesia from a test dose. For non-opioid and mixed pain we anticipate only 2–4h of good quality analgesia. This information can be used to calculate infusion regimens and bolus requirements. The conversion dose for IT morphine is 1/300 of oral morphine equivalents.

Complications

Problems are related to both the equipment and its component parts and/or to the drugs infused.

- Infection
  - Wound infections, pump pocket infections and meningitis are all possible.
  - The incidence of postoperative wound infections is the same as for any surgical procedure under similar conditions and is treated in the same way.
  - Pump pocket infections are more serious and the whole implant is at risk if not treated aggressively.
  - Meningitis is always a possibility and will usually necessitate removal of the system. However, it is possible, to aspirate CSF from the catheter via the pump side port to confirm the diagnosis and identify antibiotic sensitivities. It is also possible to inject IT antibiotics.
- CSF leak with seroma formation and/or postdural puncture headache (PDPH) is common.
- Haematomas or bleeding.
- Catheter pump disconnection.
- Gear shaft wear and motor stall. Pump stall affects 0.2% of implanted pumps 1–92 months after implant. The incidence in the USA and Canada is different from that in Europe—it is not common in Europe, except in Germany. When pumps have been returned to the manufacturer for investigation, corrosion has been evident on the metal surfaces and gears causing degradation, cracking of metal, and electrical short circuits. This is suggested to be caused by corrosive species penetrating the silicone catheter over time. Chloride, sulphur, carbon, copper, zinc, and nickel have all been identified. Compounded formulations of drugs are thought to be the culprits; those containing sodium metabisulphite are a particular problem as this compound can form sulphur dioxide gas in acidic conditions. Sodium metabisulphite is used as an antioxidant in some branded forms of injectable morphine.
- Leakage of infused drug.
- Displacement of IT catheter.
- Kinking of IT catheter.
- Catheter occlusion. Blockage of catheters is not common, with 90 cases reported in the USA and Canada 2–184 months after implant. The material obstructing the catheter has been identified as an aggregate of denatured and precipitated CSF proteins. This is thought to occur at the site where CSF and infusate interact with minimal mixing near the catheter tip and to be related to factors specific to the infusate such as a low pH or the addition of a preservative.
- IT granulomas
  - Inflammatory masses in the dura adjacent to the catheter tip have been attributed to the use of all agents, *except* fentanyl, sufentanil, and ziconotide, in implantable devices. Presenting symptoms include loss of analgesic effect and new progressive neurology.

Diagnosis is with an MRI or CT myelogram. MRI shows a hyperintense area on T_1 sections and the area enhances with gadolinium. Drug precipitates may mimic inflammatory masses.

- The majority of granulomas are associated with morphine and hydromorphone, but experimental work has shown them to be consistent with cutaneous mast cell activation rather than being mediated by opioid receptors.
- Animal work with morphine has shown that the concentration of the drug used is important rather than the actual total dose. No dogs infused with saline developed granulomas, but one of four dogs infused with 1.5mg/mL at 330µL/h (12mg morphine daily) developed a granuloma. All of four dogs were infused with 12.5mg/mL at 40µL/h (12mg/day) developed granulomas. It would seem intuitive to use the lowest concentration of drug at the highest flow.
- In the animal model, stopping the opioid leads to resolution of the inflammatory mass. In a patient there is the potential risk of long-term neurological damage and paralysis, so surgical excision of the granuloma must be considered as the first option. Early diagnosis may mean that the opioid infusion can be stopped or substituted with saline. The granuloma can be monitored for resolution clinically and with repeated MRI. Options are to remove the system and abandon the technique, to resite with a different opioid infusion regimen, or to leave *in situ* and trial ziconotide.
- MRI scanning. Information regarding MRI scanning and Medtronic pumps is available on their website (http://www.medtronic.com). The problem is that, for the Synchromed II, the magnetic field of the scanner will temporarily stop the rotor and therefore suspend drug infusion for the duration of exposure. It should restart following removal from the magnet and the pump can be interrogated afterwards to confirm this.
- Leg oedema
  - Problematic leg oedema has been described with IT opioid infusions and may necessitate cessation of therapy. Incidence in retrospective reports is variable and quoted as 6.1%, 11.7% (50/429) and 21.7% (5/23). Oedema can affect one or both legs and can be mild to severe. Previous leg oedema and venous insufficiency appear to predispose to its development. The mechanism may well be related to opioid-induced and dose-dependent vasodilation. It tends to develop 6–24 months after initiation of therapy.
  - Reduction in the infusion of opioid helps, as does leg elevation, but diuretics, elastic stockings, and compression pumps do not seem to be effective. Swelling, discoloration, and ultimately skin ulceration can occur.
- Fat necrosis is possible as a consequence of pressure from the pump which normally has to be removed and possibly resited, usually at a later date.
- Erosion through the skin may occur as a result of pressure from the pump, particularly if the patient undergoes extreme weight loss. This is common in malignancy-associated cachexia.

Implant technique

Implanting an ITDD system starts with pre-assessment of the patient for anaesthetic and other problems. MRSA swabs and blood tests should be done if appropriate. The patient should be in optimal condition. Sometimes this may mean liaising with other professionals to allow the implant to take place safely. The proposed position of the pump in the abdomen or lower chest wall should be established beforehand. The presence of stomas may limit placement. Ideally it should not be in the centre of a potential radiotherapy field.

The Medtronic implant kit for the Synchromed II comprises:
- an option of two 15G introducing needles for the dural puncture (one 9.3cm and the other 11.4cm)
- a radio-opaque silicone catheter 38cm long with a closed tip, six exit ports, and an inserted guidewire and anchor
- a proximal catheter section 66cm long that attaches to the pump and is equipped with a sutureless pump connector and a catheter–catheter connector pin and covering sleeve
- a tunnelling device
- a 20/40mL pump filled with saline.

An N-vision programmer is required and a pre-ordered refill syringe of drugs from your pharmacy aseptics unit.

It is possible to implant completely under LA, completely under general anaesthesia, or a mixture of the two. There are advantages and disadvantages to each. Ideally, the catheter can be sited under LA, as there is a finite chance of damaging the spinal cord and a conscious patient will tell you if there is a problem. However, some patients, such as children or adults with severe pain in the position required on the operating table, cannot tolerate a procedure under LA. In such cases the whole procedure can be performed under general anaesthesia. Our preferred technique for the placement of the spinal catheter is to position the patient prone and awake with a pillow under the abdomen and pelvis.

A suitable interlaminar space can be identified using a C-arm and fluoroscopy. A true AP view of the spine is needed and some cranio-caudal tilt may be necessary to square the vertebral endplates. This is often difficult to establish and maintain in a conscious patient in the lateral position. Ideally, L2/3 should be used for catheters to be passed rostrally further up the spinal canal and L4/5 or L3/4 for those going caudally to the bottom of the dural sac at S2. Anatomical/surgical factors (e.g. instrumented lumbar fusion) may necessitate puncturing the dura above the level of termination of the spinal cord at L1/2, which potentially carries more risk of spinal cord damage than puncture below. There need to be at least two vertebral spaces between dural puncture and catheter tip to fix the catheter securely.

A paramedian fluoroscopic-guided dural puncture is the safest and easiest approach, obviously from the side to which the catheter is eventually going to be tunnelled. For example, if the pump is to positioned in the right iliac fossa, a right paramedian approach is appropriate. We use 1% lidocaine with 1:200,000 adrenaline LA up to 40mL to infiltrate the proposed puncture site of skin and the track down to the lamina. A relatively shallow angle of puncture may help the catheter remain posterior rather than anterior in the spinal canal—similar to positioning of dorsal column electrodes for spinal cord stimulation. There is no way of directing a catheter currently as it has no steering, but the aim of drug infusion is to reach the dorsal horn cells that are posterior in the spinal cord. It is also necessary to anaesthetize laterally to the needle puncture site so that a small pocket can be made for the anchor and the connector.

Insert the introducing needle down to the lamina and then withdraw slightly and redirect to puncture the dura, all under X-ray screening, initially AP as far as the lamina but then a lateral view is helpful to assess the depth in the spinal canal. The puncture is often obvious with a gratifying jet of crystal-clear CSF. If the needle feels as though it ought to be correctly positioned, options are to try and establish a flow of CSF using radio-opaque dye to confirm the position initially and then a saline flush. Cold saline in a sufficiently large volume will cause an unpleasant neuropathic type pain. If there is still no CSF at this point, there is still the option to try and pass a catheter, with a default of a second dural puncture if the catheter does not pass.

Multiple dural punctures with a large-bore introducing needle run a high risk of causing a PDPH, and deferral to an open surgical technique is always worth considering.

Pass the catheter through the introducing needle under screening to the nominated vertebral level. Once the catheter is through the needle tip it is inadvisable to withdraw it as there is a risk of the catheter shearing off on the sharp bevel of the needle. The recommendation is that the whole needle–catheter unit should be withdrawn as a unit, the needle resited, and the catheter repassed. If the catheter does not pass easily—it is not possible to direct or force it—flushing with small aliquots of saline may be helpful and it is also possible to reposition the patient.

Once the catheter has been sited, withdraw the guidewire inside, check for (ideally) free flow of CSF, and confirm the position with a small aliquot of radio-opaque contrast (e.g. Ultravist 370).

Re-introduce the guidewire to minimize CSF leakage and dissect down the introducing needle to the spinal fascia. It is essential that the needle remains in place at this point to protect the catheter from damage. Also, create a small pocket lateral to the site where the needle punctures the fascia, as it is here that the anchor and connector and catheter loops will sit. Only once this is complete can the introducing needle be removed over the catheter. Do this under X-ray screening and be sure that the guidewire is partially removed first. The catheter is often inadvertently advanced rostrally during this process, so it may need readjusting once the needle has been removed. Take care not to do this excessively, as sometimes the catheter can be gripped tightly by the spinal fascia and it is not possible either to re-insert the guidewire or to withdraw the catheter.

Now that the needle has been removed, thread the anchor over the catheter. Clamp or tie the end of the catheter at this point to prevent excessive leakage of CSF. Stitch the anchor in place to clamp the catheter firmly at the site of puncture of the fascia.

If the patient is awake and prone, confirm at this point that all is well. Any pain from the catheter should have been more than obvious. If the patient is anaesthetized already, continue as described. Otherwise, either use bupivacaine intrathecally via the catheter to proceed under LA (as long as the tip is at T10 or above) or proceed after general anaesthesia.

The next steps proceed with the patient in the lateral position—right or left depending on the proposed site of the pump implant.

Now is a convenient moment (whilst the patient is being anaesthetized) to attend to the pump. The saline inside needs to be completely aspirated with the Huber (non-coring) needle provided. The drug syringes from the pharmacy can be checked and the pump refilled with these.

The next step, when the patient is in position, is to prepare the pump pocket via an incision just large enough to allow easy insertion of the pump. Then dissect down to the fascia overlying the muscle with the proviso that there should be no more than 5cm of subcutaneous tissue between the skin and the pump. Otherwise there may be programming problems.

The catheter which connects to the spinal catheter and the pump should be tunnelled subcutaneously (front to back) from the spinal incision to the pump pocket via the tunnelling device. Bending this aids passage. At this point there is a spinal catheter (clamped but fixed in place), a catheter from the pump pocket to the spinal wound, and a filled, but as yet unprogrammed, pump.

There is a risk of PDPH following the procedure, and at this point you can unclamp or untie the spinal catheter and replace some of the lost CSF with saline. We use 20–40mL. Too much will produce an unpleasant neuropathic pain. In addition to this, it is important to hydrate the patient both during and after the procedure, either orally or intravenously depending on the clinical situation.

You can now connect the spinal catheter to the pump catheter via the connecting device and sleeve. Small loops of catheter are useful to ease tension in the system and provide some slack in case of expansion later (e.g. ascites, organomegaly), but the spinal catheter will often need some trimming. The piece removed needs to be retained for calculating the catheter priming bolus later. The sleeve can be sutured to the fascia in the side pocket.

Once the CSF has reached the distal end of the new catheter, the catheter can be connected to the pump itself and the pump can be programmed with both a priming bolus and the nominated background infusion rate. PTM settings can be established at this point or later. It is useful to give cancer patients an additional bolus at this point to cover their 'normal' cancer pain—this may be the same bolus as that proposed for the PTM and it can be adjusted later depending on the response.

If ziconotide is used, a rather complicated 'pump-washing' procedure has to be performed as adsorption of the drug on internal device surfaces such as titanium effectively reduces the concentration in the reservoir: 2mL of 25micrograms/mL ziconotide should be used to rinse the internal pump surfaces after aspiration of the saline. This is repeated so that a total of three rinses are performed. The pump *must* be refilled in 2 weeks. After this refill times are 'as normal'. The starting rate of infusion for ziconotide is 2.4micrograms/day.

The pump can now be sited in the pocket with any excess catheter coiled in loops behind it. Ideally, the central pump port should not underlie the suture line. There are suture attachment loops on the pump. Sutures may prevent pump movement, but may also tether it in an uncomfortable position for the patient. A Dacron pouch for the pump is also available, which may prevent excessive mobility and aid encapsulation. The disadvantage of using a Dacron pouch is a reflection of its advantage—removal is a difficult and blood-soaked (if only local) procedure.

At this point the spinal catheter is *in situ* and connected to the pump, which is in place, filled with the chosen drug and going through the priming dose infusion as per the programming instructions. It is now time to suture the spinal and abdominal incisions—an absorbable fat stitch such as 3/0 vicryl is usually used and there is a choice of skin sutures or staples. There is some evidence from orthopaedics that absorbable subcuticular suturing may have a lower postoperative infection rate than staples—it is certainly more attractive to look at in the ensuing months and years!

Use Steri-Strips to close the wound edges and a transparent dressing, so that frequent dressing changes can hopefully be avoided. Wound glue is available and provides a waterproof finish. Finally, a wound block of 0.5% bupivacaine is a postoperative kindness.

A good description of operative techniques for those who are not surgically trained is included in 'Further Reading', 📖 p. 188.

Postoperative management

Postoperative management will vary according to the clinical condition of the patient and the reason for the implant. A 'fit and well' young patient with CRPS and a ziconotide infusion pump, for example, may be able to go home in a few hours, whereas an unwell cancer patient may be an inpatient for a few days as they recover from the surgery and opioid changes and learn to manage their PTM. Standard monitoring is essential, particularly for opioid- and LA-based regimens.

Enteral/transdermal opioids should rarely be stopped straight away. Our usual regimen for CP is to halve long-acting preoperatively opioids after surgery and then every 72h. It is often not possible to stop them completely, as a CP problem is frequently multifocal and multifactorial. Sometimes a previously unknown problem will come to light when the patient's 'main pain' is controlled, for example headache from cranial metastases in a patient with breast cancer and pelvic bone pain once the pelvic pain is controlled. In a patient with CNMP, rapid opioid/dose titration is not so pressing, so there is more time to increase IT drugs whilst reducing oral opioids. For patients on ziconotide, the starting dose is unlikely to be effective enough to reduce any regular medication.

Hydration is essential peri- and postoperatively. A PDPH is extremely unpleasant for the patient and can delay discharge for weeks. Blood patching is not recommended because of the risk of introducing infection and of damage to the spinal catheter. It is possible to inject saline through the side port of the pump (under X-ray screening) to relieve symptoms of a PDPH.

PTM use can be re-demonstrated, and doses and infusion rates adjusted depending on response. The patient can be discharged once comfortable and informed. Staples or non-absorbable sutures can be removed after 7 days; this is a good time for wound review.

Clear instructions regarding dose-reduction schedules must be given to the patient's usual carer. An information booklet with both general information regarding ITDD and information specific to the patient is invaluable for the patient to take with them on discharge. Other health professionals that the patient might meet should be fully informed about the drugs and doses used, the risk of infection, and MRI scanning procedure.

Infusion regimens and management post-implant

Several recommendations have been made for minimizing the potential spinal toxicity of infused drugs;

- minimizing local concentrations of drugs against neural tissue by appropriate catheter placement
- high flow rates
- using the lowest drug concentration possible and more complex dosing
- demand- or activity-based dosing
- variable flow rates
- intermittent bolus delivery.

The Polyanalgesic Consensus Conference in 2007 produced recommendations for maximum intrathecal doses and concentrations (Table 10.2).

Table 10.2 Recommendations for maximum intrathecal doses and concentrations

Drug	IT dose	Concentration
Morphine	15mg/day	20mg/mL
Hydromorphone	4mg/day	10mg/mL
Bupivacaine	30mg/day	40mg/mL
Clonidine	1.0mg/day	2.0mg/mL
Ziconotide	19.2micrograms/day	100micrograms/mL

Opioids for non-cancer pain

Opioid infusions can be titrated to effect over a period of months for non-cancer-related pain and oral/parenteral opioids can be reduced simultaneously. Rapid opioid titrations are unnecessary and could be dangerous as deaths associated with these have been reported.

It is certainly possible to add clonidine rather than increasing the opioid, particularly for neuropathic pain.

Ziconotide

The initial infusion rate is 2.4micrograms/day. The first refill must be 14 days after implant because of drug adsorption onto pump components. Subsequent refills must be at least every 40 days if diluted ziconotide is used and every 84 days for the 'neat' solution, depending on dose.

Dose increases are made in no more than 2.4micrograms increments per day at intervals of no more than 2–3 times per week. The maximum recommended dose is 19.2micrograms/day. There is obviously a trade-off between 'rapid' dose increases and side effects, and a slower titration regimen (e.g. rate increases of 1.2micrograms/day every 2 weeks) is likely to be both better tolerated and more successful.

It is safe to stop ziconotide infusions. The CSF drug level will drop to 5% of infusion concentration 24h after discontinuing treatment.

It is possible to use ziconotide in drug mixtures, but this reduces drug stability so that refills need to be more frequent—probably every 4 weeks for mixes with hydromorphone and much more frequently for LA mixes.

Local anaesethetic

The availability of 4% bupivacaine (40mg/mL) and the PTM means that this is now feasible. High background infusions of LA are rarely effective, except in the very short term, and so a very low background rate is sufficient. The bolus can be set according to effect and side effects, likewise the duration of infusion and the maximum activations per day via the PTM.

Opioid–clonidine–LA mixes

These combinations are used for pain that is partially sensitive to opioid and are particularly useful for CP.

For cancer pain we calculate infusion mixes such that ~1mL will last for a day—e.g. 2.5mg hydromorphone background infusion with a potential for 5 × 0.5mg boluses over the course of the day with a 5mg/mL concentration.

Our standard cancer pain mix is 200mg hydromorphone (5mg/mL) with 4.8mg clonidine (120micrograms/mL) made up to 40mL with 4% bupivacaine (40mg/mL). Other mixes may contain less hydromorphone and less bupivacaine.

PTM boluses

Boluses have to be titrated individually. This can be done easily using the single bolus facility on the N-vision programmer. If the patient has already had a couple of boluses as part of their test dose and in theatre during pump implantation, you will already have information on how effective x mg hydromorphone ± y mg LA will be and for how long it will last.

A maximum bolus from the 'standard cancer pain mix' is 2.5–5mg hydromorphone + 20mg LA + 60micrograms clonidine over 30min. High doses are occasionally necessary for malignant nerve root invasion/compression.

Trouble-shooting

Complications and their management have already been described, but what happens when the pump does not seem to work after previous efficacy?

The pump will reveal error logs on interrogation if they are present. It will also calculate the reservoir volume. If this is confirmed, the pump itself has been delivering the volumes for which it has been programmed.

If the reservoir volume is greater than that calculated, either the pump has stalled or the catheter is blocked. Fluoroscopy may confirm a lack of rotor arm movement. If the rotor arm is working, the catheter may be blocked. You can look at the catheter under X-ray to check for obvious kinks and you can also aspirate the side port for CSF or inject radio-opaque contrast through the side port. You should be mindful when injecting dye that the patient will receive a bolus of drug if the catheter is not blocked. If the pump is functioning, it is still worth investigating the catheter as there may be a disconnection or migration.

If the pump is working and the catheter is patent and connected, then another reason has to be sought. IT granuloma is a potential culprit if opioids are part of the infusate, and so MRI is indicated.

If the pump is functioning as programmed, the catheter is patent and connected, and there is no IT granuloma, either tolerance has developed to the drugs infused or there has been a change in the patient's condition and further investigation may be required. Disease progression is not uncommon in cancer patients, but there may still be treatment options (e.g. chemo- or radiotherapy). Ultimately the drug regimen may need to be altered by either increasing doses or changing the infusate component.

After death, the pump should to be removed before cremation or the alarm should be turned off.

Case studies

Case 1

A 45-year-old woman with haematuria loin pain syndrome was referred for pain management after nephrectomy and pelvic relocation of the remaining kidney in an effort to control pain. Depending on the outcome of pain management, removal of the remaining kidney, dialysis, and potential transplant were suggested. The patient was fit and well between episodes and was using pethidine for pain management. Trials of medication, including neuropathic pain agents, acupuncture, TENS, and coeliac plexus block, were all unsuccessful.

A test dose of 0.15mg diamorphine IT gave good pain relief for 24h during an episode of pain and a Synchromed EL pump was implanted. The initial infusate was 1mg/mL diamorphine and the initial infusion rate was 0.3mg/day. This completely controlled the patient's loin pain, although episodic haematuria persisted and does so to this day.

Following a warning regarding the interaction of diamorphine with the pump component resulting in potential pump stall, the pump mix was changed to hydromorphone at a concentration of 1mg/mL, initially running at 0.06mg/day (assuming that hydromorphone is five times more potent than diamorphine). This was insufficient, and so the rate was increased to 0.075mg/day and ultimately 0.1mg/day.

The pump was changed to a Synchromed II after 6 years with a similar infusate and rate of 0.1mg/day. Refills were every 3 months. There was no evident tolerance or ill effects.

Case 2

A 48-year-old man with Ehlers–Danlos syndrome was referred with a 2 year history of multiple fractures secondary to a bone metabolism problem of uncertain aetiology. He also had sleep apnoea with home continuous positive airways pressure and documented difficulty with intubation during previous anaesthetics. At the time of referral, his pain was managed with 1100micrograms/h of transdermal fentanyl with 150mg oral morphine up to hourly for breakthrough pain.

The initial management was to trial neuropathic pain medications (amitriptyline and pregabalin) with limited success. A trial of ketamine up to 100mg orally every 4h had more success, and combination enabled reduction of sevredol to 150mg every 3h.

Application for ziconotide was made without a trial because of the history of recurrent chest infections related to hypoventilation consequent on the rib fractures and a high risk of infection. A Synchromed II pump was implanted completely under LA because of anaesthetic risk. The catheter tip was sited at T7. Infusion started at 2.4micrograms/day and was increased every 14 days by 1.2micrograms/day up to 12micrograms/day.

A pre-existing lack of appetite persists, but pain is markedly better controlled. Fentanyl patches were discontinued completely and oral morphine reduced further to 30mg every 4h as required. New fractures are managed with regular oral morphine 40mg every 4h and ketamine 50mg every 4h for 2 weeks and then reduced. The course was complicated by recurrent chest infections with hypoxia, often necessitating ITU/HDU admission. The patient was wheelchair bound.

Case 3

Initial management was with an intrathecal phenol block following a test

A 36-year-old woman was referred for management of perineal pain. The pain was due to a recently formed open discharging perineal wound and a recently diagnosed recurrent progressive tumour invasion of the pelvic sidewalls. Her original diagnosis was a late presentation of a primary cervical carcinoma. She had had a pelvic exenteration 5 years previously and both chemo- and radiotherapy. Oral, transdermal, and subcutaneous opioids had not been effective, and she was on 800mg/day of oral morphine equivalents.

dose with 0.6mL of 0.5% heavy bupivacaine (3mg). Unfortunately, the phenol gave only a temporary effect. An IT test dose of 2mg hydromorphone + 30micrograms clonidine + 2mg bupivacaine was tried. The block partially effective for 90min only, compared with very good relief from a previous test dose of 3mg bupivacaine prior to the phenol block.

A Synchromed II pump was implanted with a catheter passed retrograde from L4/5 to the bottom of the dural sac at S2. An infusate of 4% bupivacaine was delivered at a background rate of 5mg/day and PTM settings of a 4mg bolus over 6min with a lockout of 2h and a maximum activation rate of 10 per day. This gave analgesia for 4–6h; the bolus was used 6–8 times per day. At the end of 2 weeks the bolus was increased to 6mg over 9min, which improved the duration and quality of analgesia. Refills were made every 4 weeks.

Further reading

Ahmed SU, Martin NM, Chang Y (2005). Patient selection and trial methods for intraspinal drug delivery for chronic pain: a national survey. *Neuromodulation* **8**: 112–20.

Bedder MD, Bedder HF (2009). Spinal cord stimulation surgical technique for the nonsurgically trained. *Neuromodulation* **2** (Suppl 1): 1–19.

Bernards CM (2006). Cerebrospinal fluid and spinal cord distribution of baclofen and bupivacaine during slow IT infusion in pigs. *Anesthesiology* **105**: 169–78.

British Pain Society (2008). *Intrathecal Drug Delivery for the Management of Pain and Spasticity in Adults: Recommendations for Best Clinical Practice*. Available online at: http://www.britishpainsociety.org/itdd_main.pdf.

Deer T, Smith HS, Cousins M, *et al.* Consensus guidelines for the selection and implantation of patients with noncancer pain for ITDD. *Pain Physician* **13**: E175–213.

Deer T, Krames ES, Hassenbusch SJ, *et al.* (2007). Polyanalgesic Consensus Conference 2007: Recommendations for the management of pain by ITDD: report of an interdisciplinary expert panel. *Neuromodulation* **10**: 300–28.

Dominguez E, Sahinler B, Bassam D, *et al.* (2002). Predictive value of IT narcotic trials for long-term therapy with ITDD in chronic non-cancer pain patients. *Pain Pract* **2**: 315–25.

Peng PW, Fedoroff I, Jacques L, Kumar K (2007). Survey of the practice of spinal cord stimulators and intrathecal analgesic implants for management of pain in Canada. *Pain Res Manag* **12**: 281–5.

Autonomic blocks

N.T. Collighan, K.N. Shoukrey, R. Munglani, S. Tordoff, L. Lynch, D. Bush, S. Das, and G. Baranidharan

Stellate ganglion/cervicothoracic sympathetic block

The stellate ganglion block is used for diagnosis and treatment of sympathetically maintained pain in the upper limbs, head, and neck and in disorders related to poor vascularity in these areas.

Indications

- Pain syndromes: CRPS, phantom limb pain, refractory angina, and post-herpetic neuralgia.
- Vascular insufficiency: Raynaud's syndrome, vasospasm, emboli, trauma, scleroderma, frostbite, and obliterative vascular disease.
- Hyperhidrosis of the upper limb.

Contraindications

- Coagulopathy
- Recent myocardial infarction
- Glaucoma
- Pneumothorax
- Pneumonectomy of the contralateral side and pathological bradycardia.

Anatomy (Fig. 11.1)

The cervical sympathetic chain is made up of the superior, middle, intermediate, and inferior cervical ganglia. The superior cervical ganglion is approximately 3–5cm long and lies on the longus capita muscle anterior to the transverse processes of C2, C3, and occasionally C4. The middle ganglion lies on the longus colli muscle anterior to the transverse process of C6; this is the smallest ganglion and is located just above the inter-mediate ganglion that lies just medial to the vertebral artery. In 80% of the population the inferior cervical ganglion is fused with the first thoracic ganglion to form the stellate ganglion (cervicothoracic ganglion). This ganglion lies anterior to the vertebral body of C7, on or above the neck of the first rib, and is ~1cm long.

Anterior to the ganglion lie the carotid sheath, the sternocleido-mastoid muscle, and skin and subcutaneous tissue. Anteriorly and inferiorly to the ganglion is the dome of the lung. Medial to the ganglion are the prevertebral fascia, the vertebral body of C7, the oesophagus, the trachea, the recurrent laryngeal nerve, and the thoracic duct. Posteriorly lie the vertebral artery as well as the longus colli muscle, the anterior scalene muscle, the brachial plexus, and the neck of the first rib.

The landmark and guide when performing the block is the anterior tubercle of C6, which is known as Chassaignac's tubercle. The ganglion lies at the level of C7, but the needle is classically inserted at the level of C6 (level with the cricoid cartilage and Chassaignac's tubercle); this reduces the risk of pleural and vertebral artery puncture. In 90% of cases the vertebral artery runs anterior to the ganglion at the level of C7 before it enters the foramen transversarum in the C6 transverse process. It must be noted that in 10% of cases the artery enters the foramen transversarum at the level of C5 and so even a C6 level block risks arterial puncture.

Arterial vessels other than the vertebral artery (e.g. the inferior thyroid vessels) may pass directly anterior to the C6 and C7 transverse processes, further increasing the risk of arterial puncture and vasospasm, haematoma, and other vascular complications.

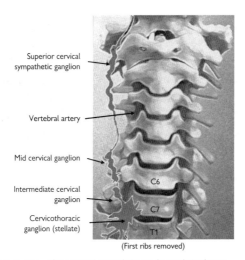

Superior cervical
sympathetic ganglion

Vertebral artery

Mid cervical ganglion

Intermediate cervical
ganglion

Cervicothoracic
ganglion (stellate)

C6

C7

T1

(First ribs removed)

Fig. 11.1 Anatomy of the cervical sympathetic ganglion and its relations.

Techniques

The location of critical structures close to the ganglion necessitates a secure technique. Blind techniques have been superseded by fluoroscopic, CT, and ultrasound guidance.

Fluoroscopic guidance

The patient lies supine with the neck supported and in slight extension. The C-arm should lie in the AP plane over the lower cervical region. The C6 and C7 vertebrae and, from these, the transverse process of C6 and Chassaignac's tubercle are identified. The point where the transverse process of C6 meets the vertebral body is marked. Choice of the medial point of the transverse process theoretically avoids the risk of a carotid artery puncture which may occur with a more laterally placed needle. Ensure that the patient is relaxed and breathing through the mouth to avoid any swallowing that may move the needle. Ensure that a method of communication with the patient is confirmed (e.g. a hand signal from the opposite side) as talking may disturb needle placement at any point of the procedure. Infiltrate 1–2mL 1% lidocaine at the marked skin point. Advance a 5cm 22G or 25G spinal needle towards the target point. The path of the needle should remain in the coaxial plane of the X-ray beam, and in the more superficial tissues a clamp may be required to hold it in position. Check this repeatedly with postero-anterior (PA) images during slow intermittent 2–4mm needle advancements. The needle should remain perpendicular to the operating table in all planes. The endpoint is contact with the bony transverse process, usually at a depth of 2–2.5cm (Fig. 11.2). The needle should then be withdrawn ~2–3mm to ensure that the tip lies outside the longus colli muscle.

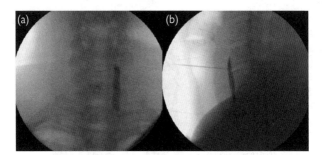

Fig. 11.2 (a) PA and (b) lateral radiographs showing needle placement at the C6 level at the junction of the transverse process and the vertebral body.

Once *in situ*, the needle tip position is checked and intravascular/intrathecal placement is ruled out by injection of 1–1.5mL radio-opaque contrast medium (e.g. Iohexhol 180mg/mL). PA and lateral X-rays should show cephalad and caudal spread of the contrast medium along the anterolateral margins of the vertebral bodies. If the tip is intra-vascular, the contrast will rapidly dissipate. If the tip is in the longus colli the cephalad/caudal spread will be restricted.

Correct positioning of the needle must be confirmed before further injection of therapeutic substances. A standard therapeutic substance is 10–20mL bupivacaine 0.125–0.25% ± 8mg dexamethasone. This is advised as it is the least particulate of the steroids available and there is theoretically less embolic and obstructive risk if accidental intravascular injection occurs. Vasospasm may still occur. A test dose of 0.5–1mL should be injected to check for intravascular injection. The patient should be monitored to ensure that there are no adverse effects. Following this, the injectate should be administered in 3–4mL aliquots with repeat radiographs that should show dilution and dissemination of the contrast in the cephalad and caudal direction, including over the C7/T1 level to ensure coverage of the stellate ganglion. The needle can be placed at a similar position on the C7 transverse process, but there is increased risk of puncture of the vertebral artery and the dome of the lung.

CT guidance

Using CT scanning the needle can be advanced directly towards the stellate ganglion at the level of the C7 vertebral body. CT images allow the vertebral artery and vein and the dome of the lung to be avoided. Because of the increased radiation exposure required for CT, use of this technique must be justified (e.g. difficult anatomy and previous complications). The procedure is similar to that used with fluoroscopic guidance but the needle is advanced towards the point of the border between the vertebral body of C7 and its transverse process, just inferior to the uncinate process. All the same precautions should still be followed prior to and after injection of a therapeutic substance to check for intravascular placement and other complications.

Ultrasound guidance

This technique should only be performed by clinicians proficient in ultrasound-guided interventions. The ultrasound scanning (USS) technique can be learned by performing it alongside the fluoroscopic technique.

With the patient in the standard position the USS transducer is placed at the level of the C6 vertebra and a cross-sectional image obtained at that level. The structures that should be visualized include the carotid artery, the internal jugular vein, the thyroid gland, the trachea, the oesophagus, the longus colli muscle, the root of C6, and the transverse process of C6. Gentle pressure with the transducer should deflect the carotid artery laterally and bring the longus colli muscle closer. After local infiltration, advance the needle towards the middle of the longus colli in the plane of the USS beam. The endpoint is either just before or just after penetration of the prevertebral fascia in the longus colli (studies show that spread with a subfascial injection is more extensive than with a suprafascial injection, but neither covered the stellate ganglion!). Precautions must always be taken to check for incorrect needle placement before titrated injection of the therapeutic substance.

Indications of a correctly placed stellate ganglion block
- Increase in the temperature of the ipsilateral limb by 1°C
- Venodilation of the ipsilateral limb
- Horner's syndrome (miosis, ptosis, and enopthalmos)
- Anhidrosis
- Nasal congestion

Complications

Technique-related
- Intravascular needle placement and injection causing haematoma, haemothorax, seizure, or vascular occlusion leading to stroke and paralysis.
- Trauma to the vertebral artery, carotid artery, internal jugular vein, and other vessels.
- Neural injury including the dorsal root, vagus nerve, and brachial plexus.
- Pneumothorax and pulmonary injury.
- Chylothorax following thoracic duct injury.
- Mediastinitis following oesophageal perforation.
- Abscesses with soft tissue infection.
- Meningitis.
- Osteitis.

Pharmacological
- Intravascular injection of LA may cause seizure, stroke, or paralysis depending upon which vessel is penetrated.
- Intrathecal spread, epidural spread, or brachial plexus blockade.
- Hoarseness (recurrent laryngeal nerve blockade) or an elevated hemidiaphragm (phrenic nerve blockade).

Horner's syndrome indicates a successful block of the face.

Thoracic sympathetic chain blockade

Introduction

Thoracic sympathetic ganglion block is a technique that can produce dramatic relief for patients suffering from certain types of pain. The proximity to the spinal cord and exiting nerve roots and pleura makes it imperative that this procedure is carried out only by someone who is well versed in the regional anatomy and experienced in interventional pain management techniques.

Anatomy

The thoracic pre-ganglionic sympathetic fibres exit the intervertebral foramen with the thoracic spinal nerves with which they interface via the myelinated pre-ganglionic fibres of the white rami communicantes and the unmyelinated post-ganglionic fibres of the grey rami communicantes. The latter fibres provide sympathetic innervation to the vasculature, sweat glands, and pilomotor muscles of skin. Other thoracic sympathetic post-ganglionic fibres travel to the cardiac plexus and course up and down the sympathetic trunk to terminate in distant ganglia.

The first sympathetic ganglion fuses with the lower cervical ganglion to form the stellate ganglion. The upper thoracic ganglia lie just beneath the rib but the lower thoracic ganglia lie more anterior to the rest along the posterolateral surface of the vertebral body. The pleural space lies lateral and anterior to the thoracic sympathetic chain. Because of the close relationship of the thoracic somatic nerves to the thoracic sympathetic chain, the potential exists for both neural pathways to be blocked during blockade of the thoracic sympathetic ganglion (Fig. 11.3).

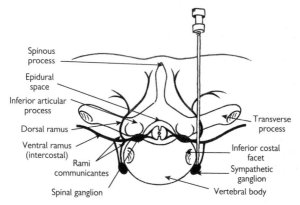

Spinous process
Epidural space
Inferior articular process
Dorsal ramus
Ventral ramus (intercostal)
Rami communicantes
Spinal ganglion
Transverse process
Inferior costal facet
Sympathetic ganglion
Vertebral body

Fig. 11.3 Needle placement for thoracic sympathetic ganglion block.

Indications

- Evaluation and management of sympathetically mediated pain of the upper thorax, chest wall, and thoracic and upper abdominal viscera.
- Diagnostic tool when performing differential neural blockade on anatomical basis for evaluation of chest, thoracic, and upper abdominal pain.
- Indicator of the degree of pain relief that a patient may experience if destruction of the thoracic sympathetic chain is being considered.
- Post-thoracotomy pain, acute herpes zoster, post-herpetic neuralgia, and phantom breast pain after mastectomy.
- Destruction of the thoracic sympathetic chain is indicated for palliation of pain syndromes that have responded to thoracic sympathetic blockade with LAs. This is often used in cancer-related pain.

Technique

- General preparations for any invasive procedure, including assessment, preparation, and patient consent (📖 Chapter 3, p. 24), are followed.
- The patient is placed in the prone position with a pillow under the lower chest to flex the thoracic spine slightly.
- Fluoroscopy is used to identify the level intended to block.
- The spinous process of the vertebra just above the nerve to be blocked is palpated
- The skin at a point just below and 5–6cm lateral to the spinous process is prepared with antiseptic solution.
- A 22G 8cm needle is advanced perpendicular to the skin, aiming para-vertebrally and inferior to the transverse process.
- If the needle impinges on the lateral margin of the vertebra it should be withdrawn and directed more laterally, staying as medial as possible (i.e. paravertebral). The needle is aimed to make contact with the transverse process, and then it is redirected inferiorly and walked off the inferior margin of the transverse process.
- A lateral X-ray view is needed as the needle is then advanced very slowly until the junction of the posterior third and anterior two-thirds of the vertebral body is reached (Fig. 11.4). To reach this point the intervertebral foramen is crossed and the spinal root may be contacted. If paraesthesiae are elicited, reposition the needle either more caudal or more cephalad and continue to advance, staying as paravertebral as possible. Do not advance beyond the midpoint of the vertebral body on the lateral view as the risk of pneumothorax increases.
- After aspiration reveals no blood or CSF, 5mL of 1.0% lidocaine or 2–2.5mL levobupivacaine 0.5% are injected. If there is an inflammatory component to the pain, the LA is combined with a steroid.
- If RF lesioning is being considered, two or three 90° 60s lesions are performed after appropriate motor stimulation to exclude proximity to the spinal root (2–3Hz at 2V) and, if possible, pain is reproduced by stimulation at 50Hz and 0.5V.

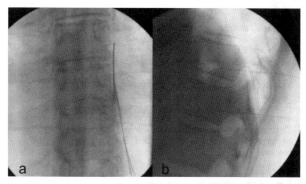

Fig. 11.4 (a) AP view of needle placement for thoracic sympathetic nerve block Notice how the needle is kept as paravertebral as possible (this reduces the risk of a pneumothorax). (b) Ideal positioning for thoracic sympathetic chain blockade with LA or RF lesioning. If the needle is placed too anteriorly, the risk of pneumothorax increases.

Complications
- Pneumothorax is a possibility given the close proximity of the pleural space. The incidence will be decreased if care is taken to keep the needle placed medially against the vertebral body. A curved tipped needle can be very helpful in keeping the needle close to the vertebral body.
- Epidural, subdural, or subarachnoid injection and trauma to the spinal cord and exiting nerve roots can result if the needle is placed too medially.
- Infection, although uncommon, is a possibility, especially in immunocompromised patients. Early detection is crucial to avoid potentially life-threatening sequelae.

Clinical pearls of wisdom
- Given the proximity of the thoracic sympathetic chain to the somatic nerve, paraesthesiae may be elicited in the distribution of the corresponding thoracic paravertebral nerve. If this occurs, the needle should be withdrawn and redirected slightly more cephalad, care being taken to keep the needle close to the vertebral body to avoid pneumo-thorax.
- Neurolytic sympathetic block with even small volumes of phenol in glycerine is not recommended as the solution can spread to the spinal roots. RF lesioning may provide longer-term relief from sympathetically mediated pain that has been relieved with LA. There is only a small risk of increasing pain with this technique (<5%).

Splanchnic nerve ablation with radio-frequency lesioning

Introduction

The management of chronic abdominal pain presents a considerable clinical challenge for pain clinicians. It is essential to establish a cause, but this might not be evident in many clinical situations. The management of chronic abdominal pain requires a multidisciplinary approach using a bio-psychosocial model. Therapeutic options involve the use of analgesics, medications for neuropathic pain, interventional nerve blocks, and complementary therapies. It is also important to consider psychological factors that might be contributing to the clinical problem.

Anatomy

The splanchnic nerves consist of three branches known as the greater, lesser, and least splanchnic nerves. They supply autonomic and sensory innervation to the abdominal organs, and contain pre-ganglionic sympathetic and afferent visceral fibres. They are extensions of the sympathetic chain that runs down through the thorax, and they wrap around the body of T12 (although the anatomical position can be variable) before running on to the coeliac plexus that lies around the mesenteric artery at the level of the body of L1.

Patient selection and therapeutic goals

The therapeutic intention of ablating the splanchnic nerves is to relieve chronic abdominal pain that might be arising from the visceral organs and retroperitoneal space. It is not effective in relieving pain arising from the abdominal or lower thoracic wall.

The therapeutic goal is to reduce the level and intensity of the pain, which might allow a patient to reduce their reliance on analgesic medication and improve their quality of life.

It is essential that both the patient and the treating physician have a realistic expectation regarding the therapeutic goal of the procedure. It is not indicated in those patients who have a large psychological component to their abdominal pain or who show abnormal illness behaviours and are dependent on strong opioids. These patients should not undergo the procedure, and pain-management strategies should be focused on psychological measures and medication reduction programmes.

Contraindications

Absolute

- Patient unwilling or unable to consent to the procedure.
- Evidence of any untreated systemic infection or infection at the site of the injection.
- Patient with a coagulopathy or using anticoagulant therapy that carries a high risk of bleeding.

Relative

- Distortion of the thoracolumbar spine or derangements of adjacent anatomical structures which might make the procedure technically difficult.

- Pacemaker.
- Coexisting respiratory or cardiovascular disease which might affect the safe conduct of the procedure.
- Unrealistic expectations regarding the clinical outcome of the procedure.

Preliminary procedures

History

A thorough medical and surgical history must be obtained. This is to establish that the abdominal pain has a visceral origin and that all therapeutic options for treating the underlying cause have been considered.

Examination

A clinical examination should exclude any infection or anatomical tenderness which suggests that the pain might be arising from the abdominal wall. Examination must also exclude any signs of cardiovascular or respiratory compromise, and the patient should be assessed to ascertain whether the procedure will be technically possible (e.g. it might be inappropriate to carry out the procedure in patients who have spinal deformities or who are morbidly obese).

Investigations

A full blood count and clotting screen must be carried out in patients who are considered at risk of excessive bleeding.

Informed consent

Patients must be provided with a clear explanation of the procedure and its therapeutic goals, as well as the possible risks. The discussion of the risks must include the following.

- Infection—this is present for any interventional procedure that is carried out, and it is mandatory that the procedure is carried out with a full aseptic technique in a theatre setting.
- Bleeding— risk of puncturing the vascular structures adjacent to the nerves as well as the major vascular structures within the abdomen.
- Nerve damage— risk of damaging the root of the 12th intercostal nerve which can result in pain radiating round the side of the chest wall.
- Lung puncture–a risk of pneumothorax.
- Diarrhoea—the splanchnic nerves are pre-ganglionic fibres of the sympathetic chain, and ablation of these can induce parasympathetic overactivity resulting in increased intestinal activity and diarrhoea.
- Postural hypotension—the sympathetic ganglion blockade effect of the ablation can induce peripheral dilation and subsequent hypotension. This is aggravated in the upright position and can take up to a week to resolve.
- Pain after the procedure—the RF procedure can induce localized pain in the thoracolumbar spine immediately after the procedure and this can last for up to 10 days. The pain is musculoskeletal in nature and might be different from the abdominal pain that the patient might have experienced previously.

Technique
Preparation and monitoring
Intravenous access must be established and intravenous fluid administered to prevent hypotension during and after the procedure. The patient must be given supplementary oxygen, and the cardiovascular and ventilatory function must be monitored throughout the procedure.

Equipment
The use of fluoroscopy is mandatory. Use of a C-arm fluoroscope will allow for angulation of the X-ray beam at various angles for optimal visualization of the spine. All operating theatre personnel must wear radiation protection, and the images obtained during the procedure must be recorded. Contrast will be required to confirm the site of needle placement.

An RF lesion generator displaying impedance, voltage, current, and temperature is required. The generator must be earthed with a dispersive plate attached to the patient, and a supply of insulated 22G needles 150mm long with a 10mm exposed tip must be available (20G needles can also be used).

Positioning
The patient is placed in the prone position on the operating table. A pillow is placed under the head and chest, with another under the pelvis to extend the lumbar spine. The patient must lie so that the end of the table lies at the level of the middle of their shins; another pillow is placed under the shins for comfort. The diathermy pad is attached to the thigh and the lead is tucked up under the patient to avoid it getting in the way when the C-arm is rotated laterally.

Target identification
The target is the T12 lumbar vertebral body. This can be identified by locating the 12th rib that lies adjacent to the vertebral body, or by counting the lumbar vertebral bodies upwards from L5. Care must be taken in patients with lumbarized or sacralized vertebrae to ensure accurate localization of T12. The spinous process of T11 appears as a teardrop lying over the body of T12.

The T12 vertebral body must be 'squared off' so that there are no double endplates. A marker is placed lengthways on the patient's back, and the flat base of the image intensifier is adjusted to lie parallel with the marker (Fig. 11.5). The position of the T11 spinous process is then marked, and the marker is left lying on this point to act as a guide when the image intensifier is rotated in the coronal axis.

It is easiest for right-handed people to stand on the left-hand side of the patient and to carry out the procedure first on the right side. The C-arm is rotated on the coronal axis 25° to the right from the vertical PA position. The trick is to get the facet joints of the spine lying in the centre of the vertebral bodies (Fig. 11.6); this will provide the correct angle of approach. The diaphragm appears dark and the adjacent lung above is white. This makes an 'arrow; that runs down to the lateral edge of the vertebral body—this arrow points to the target site.

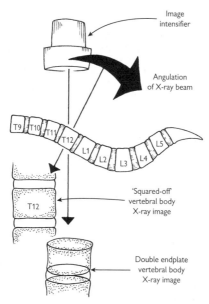

Fig. 11.5 Squaring of T12.

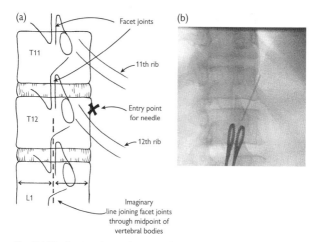

Fig. 11.6 The facet joint lying in the centre of the vertebral body and the target indicated.

Needle placement

The needle entry point is above the 12th rib at the edge of the lateral border of the body of the 12th vertebra, about a third of the way down the vertebral body (Fig. 11.6). Use a metallic marker to confirm the position. Mark this point and infiltrate the skin with LA.

The neurotomy needle must be insulated. It can be 20G or 22G and should be 150mm long with a 10mm exposed tip with an angled or coudé tip. This angulation allows the direction of the needle to be changed simply by rotating the needle on its long axis. A 'gun-barrel' technique under X-ray control is used to direct the neurotomy needle down to strike the body of the T12 vertebra. The hub of the needle is then rotated by 180° from the position at which it struck the bone in order to slide it along the vertebral body for 1cm. The needle should then be rotated 180° back again so that it lies against the bone and therefore hugs the vertebral body.

The position of the needle is then checked by fluoroscopy using a 90° AP X-ray view. The needle should lie behind the circle of the pedicle and the tip must not extend past an imaginary line that runs down the medial border of the vertebral pedicles (Fig. 11.7). The needle position should then be checked with fluoroscopy using a lateral view; the needle tip should lie in the middle third and upper anterior quadrant of the vertebral body (Fig. 11.8). A small quantity (0.5mL) of radio-opaque contrast is injected to confirm needle placement; it should outline the anterior margins of the vertebral column. The needle and contact position should be screened again to confirm the presence of the dye and to reduce the risk of intravenous placement of the needle.

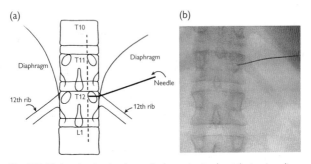

Fig. 11.7 AP view showing that the needle does not extend past the imaginary line that runs down the medial border of the vertebral pedicles.

(a)

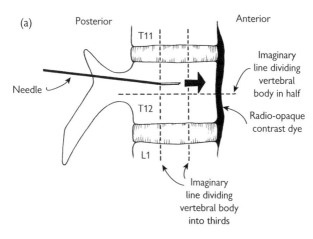

(b)

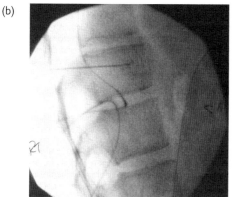

Fig. 11.8 Needle tip in the middle third and upper anterior quadrant of the vertebral body.

RF lesioning

Once the needle has been correctly positioned, a 10mL bolus of L-bupivacaine 0.5% can be injected with intermittent aspirations to reduce the risk of intravenous administration. The impedance must be checked, and must be <250Ω. The RF lesion is made by gradually increasing the temperature of the needle tip to 80°C and maintaining this for 60s. The temperature must increase in a smooth and regular manner. Fluctuations in temperature increase suggest that the needle may be lying intravascularly or in the tendon of the diaphragm. The needle is then rotated 180° on its long axis and advanced by 5mm, and the RF lesion is repeated in the same manner. The needle is again rotated 180° and advanced another 5mm, and the lesion is repeated. A total of four lesions are carried out in this way. On completion of the procedure, the needle is withdrawn 15mm and a depot preparation of steroid (methylprednisolone 60mg) is injected before withdrawing the needle.

It is imperative that the lesions are carried out when the needle has been advanced forwards towards the anterior part of the vertebral body. This will ensure that the lesions cover the area where the splanchnic nerves would be expected to lie. This reduces the risk of damaging the 12th intercostal nerve which might cause neuralgia of the lateral abdominal wall.

The procedure is repeated on the opposite side if the intention is to carry out a bilateral ablation. The C-arm is rotated to the midline position to check the level of the 12th vertebral body, and then further rotated to a 25° angle on the left side. The right-handed operator should remain on the left side of the patient, but sitting down makes it easier for some operators to adjust for the altered angle of operation that is required to carry out this procedure on the left-hand side.

Post-procedural care

Monitoring

The patient's cardiovascular and ventilatory function must be monitored. The presence of a pneumothorax must be excluded before discharge. This involves routine monitoring of the respiratory rate and vital signs, with clinical examination and auscultation of the lungs to confirm adequate and equal air entry. A sitting exhalation AP chest X-ray is mandatory and the image must be checked by the operating physician before the patient is discharged. If there are any concerns that a pneumothorax might be present, then the patient must be admitted for clinical observation for the next 12–24 hours.

Pain following the procedure

Patients must be advised that after the procedure they might experience pain in the thoracolumbar region that is different in nature to their usual abdominal visceral pain. The splanchnic nerves lie over the vertebral bodies and the RF ablation involves burning these at a temperature of 80°C. The underlying periosteum will be affected and this 'bone pain' can last for up to 10–14 days after the procedure. A patient might become distressed with both the pain and the worry that the procedure has gone wrong. Explanation and reassurance about this before the procedure usually avoids this problem. This pain responds well to simple analgesia and NSAID medication.

Medication reduction

Patients should be advised to continue with their regular medications after the procedure. They should be advised to reduce their medications gradually if they feel that their pain is reduced or better controlled. Many patients will be taking opioid medication for pain management, and they should be cautioned about reducing this too abruptly because of the risk of opioid withdrawal.

Evaluation

Clinical review

This is usually carried out 4 weeks after the procedure. An assessment of pain relief and the percentage reduction in pain is made. A discussion and explanation can be given regarding how long the block might last and when it might be repeated. Advice can also be given regarding any adjustments that need to be made to the patient's medications.

Duration of relief

This is always difficult to predict. It is inadvisable to repeat a splanchnic nerve block within 3 months of doing a previous block. Nerves that have undergone ablation with RF recover over time; this can take 9–12 months. It should be explained to patients that regeneration of the ablated nerves will occur. It is our practice to offer to schedule patients to have a repeat of the nerve ablation procedure after ~9 months, and this usually works well. The procedure can be deferred if the patient feels that it is not required after this time. Some patients will ask for the procedure to be repeated at an earlier stage.

Pearls of wisdom

It is mandatory for all patients to be clinically examined and have a chest X-ray to exclude a pneumothorax following the procedure. It has been our practice to do this and then discharge the patient home with clear instructions and information about seeking medical advice if they become unwell in the 24h following the procedure. Clinicians may feel uncomfortable doing this, and a period of observation in hospital for 12–24h following the procedure is reasonable. Patients should avoid flying or scuba diving for 7 days post-procedure.

There is no limit to the number of ablations that can be carried out on patients. The intervals between procedures should be as long as possible, given their clinical symptoms, and a balance must be struck between achieving acceptable pain management and minimizing the risks of the procedure to the patient.

In our experience many patients are unwilling to have this procedure done without any form of sedation. If they are able to manage this, they are unlikely to have a repeat procedure without sedation. Many of the textbooks describe stimulating the splanchnic nerves for concordance with the pain that the patient describes. We have tried this and have found it very difficult for both operator and patient, and it has not contributed anything of value to the procedure. If anything, it has been counterproductive and has left all parties feeling that the procedure has been unsuccessful. Our practice is to sedate the patient with an intermittent intravenous bolus of propofol. This makes the procedure acceptable for the patient and much easier for the operator because the patient stays still, allowing quick and accurate needle placement.

In practical terms we have found no clinical benefit in carrying out an LA test block, and we proceed directly to an ablation procedure after obtaining informed consent. This is because control blocks are often of short duration and are not always replicated by the ablation procedure, and the patient is exposed to a reduced risk of complications by carrying out the ablation as an initial procedure.

Some physicians recommend that the needle position must be confirmed by stimulation to obtain concordance with the patient's pain before carrying out the ablation procedure. A patient must be cooperative and communicative to achieve clinical concordance, and this is often difficult. Many patients find the procedure painful and unpleasant, and we have found this concordance difficult to achieve and it has not improved clinical outcomes. The whole procedure becomes technically difficult in patients who are moving and the risks of complications are greatly increased. Many patients are fearful of being aware during the procedure, and our practice is to administer intravenous sedation. We rely on the anatomical and radiological landmarks to ensure that the needle is correctly placed before carrying out the nerve ablations.

Will it work and how long will it work for?

These are the two questions that patients will invariably ask. We always answer 'I don't know' to each question and then go on to explain the answer. The intervention is done initially for both diagnostic and therapeutic reasons. It is our experience that some patients appear to be good candidates but then do not obtain any significant clinical benefits following the procedure, and this should be explained to them. It is important to establish realistic expectations regarding the therapeutic goals of the procedure. We explain that a good clinical result from our perspective would be if we could reduce their pain by 30% or more which might allow them to reduce their medication requirements and improve their quality of life. We also explain that this benefit might be achieved for a reasonable length of time that might be 3 months or more, and under these circumstances it would be justified to consider repeating the procedure at intervals. We explain that ablation of the nerves with RF can provide a more prolonged clinical benefit and that the regeneration of these nerves takes about 9–12 months, and this should dictate when the procedure might require repeating.

Beware of desperate patients and desperate doctors! We see many patients who have been referred for 'a block that's going to fix my problem', and we receive many referrals from colleagues who have tried everything and are at their wits' end in dealing with patients who have a long history of abdominal pain, opioid misuse, and repeated hospital admissions. These patients will not benefit from this procedure, and in our opinion it is far more important to identify those patients who will not benefit from the procedure rather than those who might.

Coeliac plexus block

Neurolytic coeliac plexus blocks (CPBs) were first described by Kappis in 1914 for the management of terminal pancreatic cancer pain. Blocks of the coeliac axis also have a role in the management of chronic abdominal pain caused by a multitude of abdominal visceral conditions. It is possible to block the splanchnic nerves before they join the coeliac plexus, the plexus itself, or the upper lumbar sympathetic chain. A variety of techniques can be used, ranging from a surgical thoracoscopic splanchnectomy under direct vision to percutaneous needle techniques under fluoroscopic screening/CT/US or via upper GI endoscopy and ultrasound guidance. The approach is normally posterior, but anterior approaches have been described. Solutions used include LA, steroids, ammonium nitrate, alcohol, and phenol. RF lesioning is an option for the splanchnic nerves, as are neuromodulation techniques using implanted electrodes.

A meta-analysis of neurolytic CPBs for the treatment of cancer pain conducted in 1995 calculated that they were effective in 70–90% patients at 2 weeks post-block and the results were maintained at 3 months.

Anatomy

The anatomy of the coeliac plexus is not entirely straightforward, which explains why many techniques have been described, why 'failures' are common, and why knowledge of anatomy can help in developing alternative strategies.

The coeliac plexus lies within the retroperitoneal space at the level of the last thoracic vertebra and the upper part of the first lumbar vertebra. A dense network of nerve fibres surrounds the coeliac artery and the root of the superior mesenteric artery and unites to form (usually) two large coeliac ganglia. It lies posterior to the stomach and the omental bursa, anterior to the crura of the diaphragm and the commencement of the abdominal aorta, and between the suprarenal glands. The plexus and the ganglia are formed by the pre-ganglionic sympathetic fibres of the greater, lesser, and least splanchnic nerves of both sides, some pre-ganglionic parasympathetic fibres from the vagus nerve, and some sensory fibres from the phrenic nerves. After synapsing in the coeliac ganglia, post-ganglionic fibres extend as numerous secondary plexuses along the neighbouring arteries. There are also contributions from the upper two lumbar sympathetic nerves which pass both up to the ganglia and directly to the secondary plexuses.

The secondary plexuses related to the coeliac are the phrenic, splenic, hepatic, left gastric, intermesenteric, suprarenal, renal, testicular or ovarian, superior mesenteric, and inferior mesenteric.

The greater splanchnic nerve consists of myelinated, pre-ganglionic, and visceral afferent fibres. It is formed by branches from the 5th to the 9th or 10th thoracic ganglia, but fibres as high as from the first thoracic ganglion have been identified. It descends obliquely on the bodies of the thoracic vertebra and perforates the crus of the diaphragm to join the coeliac plexus. Some fibres join the aortico-renal ganglion and the suprarenal gland.

The lesser splanchnic nerve is formed from the 9th and 10th or 10th and 11th thoracic ganglia. It pierces the diaphragm with the greater nerve and joins the aortico-renal ganglion.

The lowest or least splanchnic nerve arises from the last thoracic ganglion and accompanies the sympathetic trunk into the abdomen to join the renal plexus.

The upper two lumbar splanchnic nerves pass from the lumbar sympathetic ganglia to the coeliac and secondary plexuses.

The afferent fibres that accompany the pre- and post-ganglionic fibres of the sympathetic system have a segmental arrangement, and it is these that are involved with the transmission of pain:

- Oesophagus (caudal part): T5–T6
- Stomach: T6–T10
- Small intestine: T9–T10
- Large intestine as far as splenic flexure: T11–L1
- Splenic flexure to rectum: L1–L2
- Liver and gall bladder: T7–T9
- Spleen: T6–T10
- Pancreas: T6–T10
- Kidney: T10–L1
- Ureter: T11–L2
- Suprarenal: T8–L1
- Testis and ovary: T10–T11.

Indications

- Cancer-related abdominal pain (e.g. pancreatic)
- Chronic visceral pain (e.g. chronic pancreatitis, polycystic renal disease.

(Anaesthesia for upper abdominal surgery with a combination of coeliac plexus and lower intercostal nerve blocks has been described.)

Contraindications

- Bleeding diathesis
- Intra-abdominal sepsis
- Bowel obstruction
- Antabuse.

Caution

- Abdominal aortic aneurysm/vascular disease
- Polycystic kidney disease
- Gastric outflow obstruction/gastric stasis
- Pleural adhesions/disease.

Complications and side effects

- Diarrhoea is common because of unopposed parasympathetic activity. It is usually transient, but rarely persistent and severe.
- Postural hypotension is common because of vasodilation of mesenteric blood vessels, but again it is usually transient. The patient must be fasted before the procedure, so intravenous rehydration is mandatory during the procedure.

- Permanent paraplegia is reported historically as 1 in 683 posterior percutaneous CPBs. It is thought to be related to the close anatomical proximity of the artery of Adamkiewicz which supplies the anterior spinal artery of the lower third of the spinal cord. It has been suggested that more anterior approaches may reduce the incidence substantially.
- Gastroparesis.
- Diaphragmatic paralysis.
- Phrenic nerve palsy.
- Pneumothorax.
- Chylothorax.
- Retroperitoneal haematoma: the aorta is intimately related to the coeliac axis and puncture may occur in a third of patients. An intentionally trans-aortic technique has been described. The inferior vena cava is close to the right of the axis. Back pain after a block may be the first indication of this, although there are many other explanations including local bruising.
- Renal damage/haematuria.
- Aortic pseudo-aneurysm.
- Aortic dissection.
- Sexual dysfunction.

Techniques

The success of coeliac axis blockade depends on adequate spread of the chosen injectate particulary if an anterocrural technique is used. A single-needle technique may be sufficient for many non-cancer patients if tissue planes are 'normal'. Infiltration and/or compression by tumour, distortion, and/or fibrosis after surgery or inflammation and the after-effects of radio- or chemotherapy can alter tissue planes substantially. A single-needle technique is probably not going to be sufficient for this group of patients and a 'ring-block' around the axis may be necessary. Retrocrural splanchnic nerve blocks rely far less on spread of solution.

The procedure can be painful even with good LA, and sedation, sometimes heavy, is usually necessary. Intravenous fluids are also required, as the patient will have both fasted for the procedure and be prone to postural hypotension and diarrhoea afterwards.

Percutaneous blocks under fluoroscopy are the most commonly performed techniques and may be either retrocrural at T12 or anterocrural in front of L1. Several techniques have been described. The terms splanchnic and coeliac blocks are sometimes used interchangeably, but obviously the splanchnic blocks affect only the pre-ganglionic sympathetic fibres of the three splanchnic nerves and the coeliac blocks include post-ganglionic sympathetic fibres from these nerves as well as the contributions from the vagus and phrenic nerves and the upper lumbar sympathetics.

Retrocrural splanchnic nerve block

The patient is positioned prone with a pillow under the abdomen. Identify T12 with a true AP view and square off the vertebral endplates. The vertebral body of T12 lies just underneath the spinous process of T11. Tilt the C-arm approximately 20° towards the relevant side so that the facet joints lie in the middle of the vertebral bodies. Identify the 12th rib and note the triangle formed by the upper border of the rib and the anterior and superior margins of the vertebral body. Identify a point within the triangle and infiltrate the skin and subcutaneous tissues with LA. A 15cm 22G needle with a bent tip is ideal for the block. Using a gun-barrel approach aim to touch the vertebral body with the needle bent towards the bone so that a 180° rotation will enable one to slide the needle off the bone easily and advance further if necessary. When the needle touches bone, go to a lateral X-ray view. One is aiming for the upper half of the vertebral body in the middle and anterior thirds, which is where the splanchnic nerves cross the vertebra on their way through the diaphragm.

Radio-opaque contrast will confirm the position on each side. A relatively small volume of solution is required—up to 10mL of LA ± steroid, or 6mL of phenol or absolute alcohol for a neurolytic block.

There is a risk of pneumothorax with the technique, so a post-procedural X-ray is required.

Anterocrural coeliac plexus block

Positioning is similar to that for the retrocrural block with the patient prone and a pillow under the abdomen. There is no visible endpoint to aim for on fluoroscopy with this technique which aims to place either one needle anterior to the aorta in the region of the coeliac axis or one needle on either side of it. Aortic puncture probably occurs in a third of patients who have a left-sided procedure as the aorta lies to the left of the midline (AOL = aorta on left).

A single-needle technique may suffice for non-cancer pain, particularly if pain is unilateral, as the solution injected will spread along normal tissue planes quite easily. Cancer pain patients with extensive changes related to tumour, surgery, fibrosis, lymphadenopathy, radiotherapy and chemotherapy may need a different approach as the tissue planes have been destroyed. A ring-block technique around the coeliac axis may be more effective with needles on either side of the aorta anteriorly and posteriorly in a bilateral high-lumbar sympathetic block at the antero-lateral borders of L1.

The procedure begins by identifying L1. A true AP fluoroscopic view is required with the vertebral endplates squared off. Skin and deeper tissues are infiltrated with LA a hand's breadth (<10cm) from the midline after fluoroscopic screening has identified the inferior borders of the 12th rib. A long 22G spinal needle is directed under fluoroscopic guidance to touch the border of L1, avoiding the transverse process. It can then be withdrawn and redirected to 2–3cm anterior to the anterior border under a lateral fluoroscopic view. The needle stylet is withdrawn during this process—if the needle punctures the aorta it can be advanced through the lumen which should position it perfectly at the site of the coeliac axis at the other side. Radio-opaque contrast confirms the needle position.

Alternatively, after squaring the L1 vertebral endplate, an oblique view is obtained to align the transverse process of L1 with the anterior L1 body (Fig. 11.9(a)). A needle puncture point is chosen just lateral or inferior to the transverse process and an 18G needle is directed to the lateral border of the L1 body. This is advanced to a desirable depth based on the patient's body habitus using a tunnel vision technique (~5cm in a thin individual). A 22G 150mm needle (bent 1 inch at the tip) is then advanced via the 18G needle to touch the vertebral body, with the bent tip facing the vertebral body. This needle is then pulled back and rotated through180° so that the curvature is facing outside. After advancing for 1 inch, it is again rotated through 180° to hug the vertebral body (Fig. 11.9(b)). Lateral and AP views are obtained to confirm the needle-tip position just anterior to the L1 vertebral body (Fig. 11.10). Low-volume tubing is attached to the 22G needle and contrast is injected under continuous fluoroscopic view, followed by the therapeutic agent. This is to prevent accidental needle-tip movement on connecting and disconnecting at the needle hub.

Large volumes are needed—up to 50mL to obtain good spread whatever technique is used. Neurolytic blocks use 25mL of absolute alcohol and 25mL of LA. Sedation may need to be supplemented with a short-acting opioid during injection of the alcohol which is often very painful. It is probably best to keep the patient prone after a neurolytic block to help prevent the alcohol solution from spreading posteriorly.

CT guidance allows the interventional radiologist to identify the best puncture site on the skin, plot the appropriate depth and inclination of the needle, and avoid passing through the pleura and vessels. Correct needle-tip position can be confirmed and the spread of the injectate can be visualized.

Endoscopic ultrasound-guided (EUS) CPB offers an anterior approach to the coeliac axis through the posterior stomach wall, thereby avoiding the major blood vessels, diaphragm, and pleura. It couples a HF ultrasound probe and an oblique viewing endoscope utilizing real-time imaging and colour Doppler. The image quality can be good enough to evaluate pancreatic disease and to diagnose and stage pancreatic carcinoma and pancreatic neuroendocrine neoplasia.

The patient needs to be in the left lateral position and sedated. The endoscope is used initially to pass the instrument into the stomach to the lesser curvature. The ultrasound probe can then be used to identify the aorta through the stomach wall. The coeliac artery is the first vessel arising from the aorta below the diaphragm. It may be possible to visualize the actual coeliac ganglia. Once the base of the coeliac trunk has been identified, a fine aspirate needle is passed through the biopsy channel of the scope and fixed to the Luer lock assembly. The needle is then advanced under real-time ultrasound imaging through the posterior wall of the stomach immediately adjacent and anterior to the lateral aspect of the aorta and at the level of the coeliac trunk. For a neurolytic block 5–10mL of 0.25–0.5% bupivacaine and 10–20mL of 98% dehydrated ethanol are injected.

Thoracoscopic splanchnectomy is a percutaneous procedure performed under general anaesthesia. Nerves can be divided on one or both sides with the patient in either the prone or the lateral position. The procedure uses two trocars for each side and CO_2 insufflation is used to create sufficient vision and working space. (It is not necessary to use one-lung ventilation and deflate the ipsilateral lung.) The roots of the splanchnic nerves from T5 to T12 are identified with precision video assistance and divided using cautery.

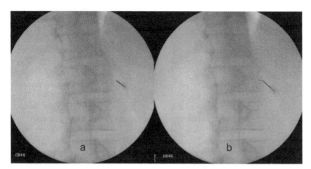

Fig. 11.9 Oblique X-ray views showing (a) 18G needle just anterior to the transverse process and (b) bent 22G needle through the 18G needle hugging the anterior vertebral body.

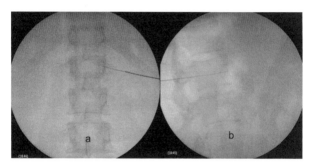

Fig. 11.10 (a) AP and (b) lateral X-ray views of the needle in the final position.

The obvious advantages of this technique are the high precision under direct vision, the avoidance of toxic chemicals, the avoidance of needle puncture of blood vessels and viscera, and no risk of paraplegia.

One of the disadvantages is the lack of effect on the upper lumbar sympathetic nerves, although this can be addressed separately. The need for general anaesthesia means that some patients may not be suitable.

Surgical blocks under direct vision at laparotomy are feasible but, rather disappointingly, are reportedly less effective than percutaneous procedures.

Choice of injectate for neurolytic blocks
The choice is between ethyl alcohol and phenol, although ammonium salts have also been used.

Alcohol works by dehydration, extraction of phospholipids, cholesterol, and cerebrosides, and precipitation of mucoproteins and lipo-proteins. This results in sclerosis and separation of the myelin sheath and oedema of Schwann cells and axons. The basal lamina of the Schwann cell tube is often spared and the axon can regenerate along its previous course. Injection of the ganglion can produce cell destruction with no subsequent regeneration. Concentrations of at least 35–50% are needed to produce neurolysis, and concentrations >95% destroy all the fibres with which the injectate comes into contact, resulting in extensive fibrosis. LA is usually used in conjunction with alcohol as the alcohol-induced neuritis can be more painful than the original pain and can take up to 4 weeks to subside. Alcohol has high solubility in body fluids and distributes widely, necessitating the use of relatively high volumes compared with phenol.

The mode of action of phenol depends on its concentration: <5% causes the denaturation of proteins and >5% causes protein coagulation, non-specific segmental demyelination, and orthograde degeneration (Wallerian degeneration). Aqueous solutions are more potent than those with glycerine, but phenol is relatively insoluble in water and so solutions with concentrations >6–7% may need additional glycerine. Concentration of 6–8% are in common use. Clinically, a biphasic effect has been described, with an LA-type effect first and then neurolysis. There is much less pain than with alcohol. The neurolytic effect may take up to a week to develop and can be repeated. Systemic doses >8.5g cause convulsions with collapse of the CNS and cardiovascular system Toxicity has not been noted with >1g, so up to 10mL of up to 10% phenol is likely to be safe.

Ammonium salts in concentrations >10% produce an acute degenerative neuropathy with obliteration of C-fibres and only a very small effect on A-fibres. The attraction of ammonium salts is that their effect is solely on pain fibres, and indeed fewer neurological complications are reported, but the current view is that their efficacy is questionable.

Summary
A variety of techniques are available and each has its advantages and disadvantages. Patient factors and local availability will probably influence the technique chosen. The blocks can be combined and are repeatable.

Further reading
Brown DL (1992). *Atlas of Regional Anesthesia*. Philadelphia, PA: WB Saunders.

Chelly JE (2009). Drugs and agents used in neurolysis and fluoroscopy. In *Peripheral Nerve Blocks: A Color Atlas* (3rd edn). Philadelphia, PA: Lippincott–Williams & Wilkins.

Eisenberg E, Carr DB, Chalmers TC (1995). Neurolytic celiac plexus block for treatment of cancer pain: a meta-analysis. *Anesth Analg* **80**: 290–325.

Garcea G, Thomasset S, Berry DP, Tordoff S (2005). Percutaneous splanchnic nerve RF ablation for chronic abdominal pain. *ANZ J Surg* **75**: 640–4.

Jain P, Dutta A, Sood J (2006). Coeliac plexus blockade and neurolysis: an overview. *Indian J Anaesth* **50**: 169–77.

Loukas M, Klaassen Z, Merbs W, Tubbs RS, Gielecki J, Zurada A (2010). A review of the thoracic splanchnic nerves and celiac ganglia. *Clin Anat* **23**: 512–22.

Prasad A, Choudhry P, Kaul S, Srivastava G, Ali M (2009). Thoracoscopic splanchnicectomy as a palliative procedure for pain relief in cancer of the pancreas. *J Minim Access Surg* **5**: 37–9.

Soweid AM, Azar C (2010). Endoscopic ultrasound-guided celiac plexus neurolysis. *World J Gastrointest Endosc* **2**: 228–31.

Standring S (ed.) (2008). *Gray's Anatomy* (40th edn). Edinburgh: Churchill Livingstone.

Lumbar sympathectomy

The lumbar sympathetic chain is a target for blockade for management of chronic pain and vascular conditions. It was first described in the 1920s, and the techniques became popular for the management of chronic pain in the 1950s. Blockade may be temporary using LA or semi-permanent using neurolytic or RF lesioning.

Indications
- Management of peripheral vascular disease (e.g. distal chronic obliterative disease, atherosclerosis, and chronic vasopastic conditions such as Raynaud's disease)
- Management of neuropathic pain (e.g. CRPS, discogenic pain)
- Hyperhidrosis

Evidence

Lumbar sympathectomy can be used as a diagnostic procedure in those with sympathetically maintained pain, although this concept remains contentious. In some neuropathic pain conditions there is basic scientific evidence that post-ganglionic sympathetic efferents influence primary afferent neurons in pathological conditions. Blockade of the lumbar sympathetics may interrupt pre- and post-ganglionic sympathetic afferents and block visceral afferents from the leg accompanying the sympathetic nerves. This may explain the clinical observations of benefit in some patients with CRPS. Lumbar sympathectomy has been used in other neuropathic pain conditions such as phantom limb pain and post-herpetic neuralgia, but evidence of benefit for these indications is weak. The evidence base to support use of lumbar sympathectomy in vascular disease and discogenic pain is weak, but the technique is still used.

Anatomy

The lumbar sympathetic chain is situated over the anterolateral surface of L2 to L4. There are usually four ganglia between L1 and L5, grouped variably between individuals. They are highly variable in size and shape (5–15mm in diameter). Pre-ganglionic fibres leave the spinal cord with the spinal nerves and reach the sympathetic chain as white rami communicantes. The relevant cell bodies lie in the anterolateral spinal cord from T10 to L3. Post-ganglionic fibres leave the sympathetic ganglia via the grey rami communicantes to join the nerve plexi accompanying the iliac and femoral vessels to supply the lower limbs. The major sympathetic supply to the lower extremities is from the second and third lumbar sympathetic ganglia.

Each lumbar sympathetic chain enters the retroperitoneal space under the right and left crura at the level of L2 in approximately two-thirds of cases and more proximally in the remainder They lie between the periosteum of the vertebra posteriorly and the retroperitoneum anteriorly, and lie medial to the origin of the psoas muscles. The aorta lies anterio-medial to the left trunk and the vena cava lies anterior to the right trunk. The chain is fixed by connective tissue to lie directly over the L2/3, L3/4, and L4/5 discs, being more variable in position over the vertebral bodies. The grey and white rami communicantes pass under the attachments of the psoas muscle to reach their ganglia (Fig. 11.11).

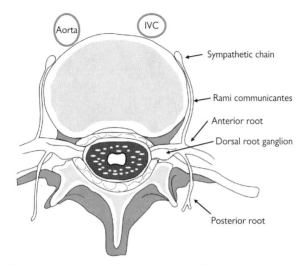

Fig. 11.11 Anatomy of the lumbar sympathetic chain: IVC, inferior vena cava. Adapted from MediClip images, copyright Alpha Media.

The position of the sympathetic chain in normal spines and in individuals with degenerative spondylophytes has been compared in a cadaver study. In the latter group the position of the sympathetic chain was more variable, bridging over the concavity of the vertebral bodies and being unpredictably displaced laterally or medially by the spondylophytes but usually remaining bound to the discs in a constant position. This suggests that blockade near discs might be more reliable in this patient group.

Technique

The patient is usually placed prone with a pillow under the abdomen to reduce lumbar lordosis, although the decubitus lateral position can be used with appropriate modification of the technique. The C-arm is centred over the mid lumbar region at L3 and rotated obliquely until the tip of the transverse process is superimposed over the anterolateral margin of the vertebra. (Fig. 11.12(a)). The optimum level for a single-needle block is the L2/3 interspace. Skin infiltration with lidocaine 1% is followed by insertion of a 22G 180mm needle that is advanced using a coaxial technique directed at the lateral margin of the L3 vertebra until it contacts bone. A curved needle tip may aid placement. Following more local anaesthesia, the needle is walked laterally off the vertebral body. The C-arm is then rotated to achieve a lateral view and the needle advanced as close to the vertebra as possible until it overlies the upper third of the vertebra (Fig. 11.12(b)). It is important to avoid trauma to the nerve root as the needle is advanced past it. Contrast (Ultravist 370) is then injected in a volume of 1–2mL. Contrast should remain applied to the antero-lateral margin of the vertebral bodies on the lateral view and remain within the vertebral margins in the AP view, indicating that the injectate is in the correct plane (Fig. 11.13).

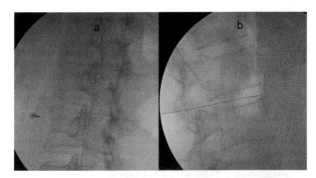

Fig. 11.12 (a) The transverse process superimposed over the anterolateral margin of the vertebra with the needle in place. (b) Lateral X-ray view of the needle position.

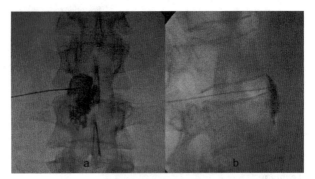

Fig. 11.13 (a) AP and (b) lateral views showing the contrast spread.

LA blockade
If an LA diagnostic or therapeutic bock is indicated, 15–20mL of LA (e.g. 0.25% bupivacaine) is injected after excluding intravascular placement by injection. One needle at L2/3 is usually sufficient for this procedure.

Confirmation of success
This can be assessed by skin temperature monitoring using pre- and post-block comparison of both limbs. A temperature rise of 2°C is taken to indicate a successful block. Change in sweating can be documented by a change in skin electrical resistance or dye testing, although this is not routine practice.

Neurolytic blockade
Neurolysis can be achieved by injecting aqueous phenol 7% which destroys nerve fibres by denaturing protein. Traditionally, three injections are made at L2, L3, and L4 using the technique already described.

Recent studies suggest that the sympathetic chain is most consistently located over the discs and so this is the preferred target site, particularly in patients with degenerative spinal disease. Often a single needle at L3 will show adequate spread of contrast from L2 to L4, obviating the need for additional injection.

RF lesioning

RF lesioning of the sympathetic ganglia can be performed by placing 15cm RF cannulae at the midpoint of L2, L3, and L4 using a technique similar to that already described. Usually 10mm active-tip electrodes are used. Sensory testing is not particularly useful. Motor stimulation can be used to exclude proximity to motor roots. Following injection of LA, RF lesions are made at 80°C for 90s. Several lesions may be required at each level.

Contraindications

The main contraindication to lumbar sympathectomy is any impairment of coagulation, as significant retroperitoneal haematoma has been reported. Sympathectomy on the same side as a unilateral kidney is a relative contraindication because of the risk of renal injury.

Complications

These should be rare with careful technique, but may include inadvertent intravascular injection of LA or neurolytic, haematuria from renal perforation, haemorrhage from puncture of a great vessel, and spinal nerve/cord injury. Spread of neurolytic onto the L1 and L2 roots can cause pain over the anterior thigh as a result of direct nerve injury. This complication should be reduced if RF is used. Bilateral neurolytic lumbar sympathectomy may be associated with immediate hypotension and long-term sexual dysfunction, particularly in males. Sexual dysfunction can also occur after unilateral block but it is rarer.

Further reading

Boas RA (1998). Sympathetic nerve blocks: in search of a role. *Reg Anesth Pain Med* **23**: 292–305.

Feigl CG, Astner MK, Ulz H, Breschan C, Dreu M, Likar R (2011). Topography of the lumbar sympathetic trunk in normal lumbar spines and spines with spondylophytes. *Br J Anaesth* **106**: 260–5.

Raj P, Lou L, Erdine S, et al. (eds) (2008). *Interventional Pain Management: Image-Guided Procedures* (2nd edn). Philadelphia, PA: WB Saunders.

Hypogastric plexus block

Introduction

Pelvic pain is often visceral, and symptoms can be vague and poorly localized compared with somatic pain. A hypogastric plexus block is useful for evaluation and management of sympathetically mediated pain of pelvic viscera. Analgesia of pelvic organs is possible because afferent fibres innervating these structures travel in sympathetic nerves via the hypogastric plexus.

Anatomy

The superior hypogastric plexus lies in front of the L5 vertebra and sacral promontory between the common iliac vessels. It is formed from fibres from the aortic plexus and splanchnic nerves, and is a continuation of the coeliac and inferior mesenteric plexus. The hypogastric nerves pass downwards, following the concave curvature of the sacrum, and then continue on each side of the rectum to form the inferior hypogastric plexus.

Viscera innervated by the superior hypogastric plexus include the bladder, uterus, vagina, prostrate, testes, urethra, descending colon, and rectum.

Indications

The hypogastric plexus block can be used for diagnostic, prognostic, or therapeutic purposes. It can be used as an adjunct to reduce analgesic consumption. It is not a panacea, given that multiple pain mechanisms that are often involved in pelvic pain.

- Malignancy (e.g. cervical, endometrial, prostrate, bladder, testis, and colorectal cancers).
- Cancer-related conditions (e.g. post-radiation cystitis, enteritis, and proctitis).
- Gynaecological problems (e.g. endometriosis, adhesions, and chronic pelvic inflammatory disease).
- Non-gynaecological problems (e.g. interstitial cystitis, irritable bowel syndrome, post-surgical chronic pain, and proctalgia fugax).

Contraindications

- Patient refusal
- Coagulopathy
- Local infection
- Sepsis
- Patient receiving radiation or chemotherapy or scheduled to receive these therapies within 4 weeks of the neurolytic block.

Technique

Equipment

A suitable room for aseptic procedure is required with a C-arm and radiological table to achieve very oblique angles (using an ordinary theatre table may be difficult).

Posterior approach

- Prone position with a pillow under the pelvis to flatten the lumbar lordosis.
- Identify the L5/S1 interspace and square the vertebral endplates using a cephalic tilt.
- Obtain an oblique view to align the transverse process of L5 with the anterior L5 body (see Figs. 11.9 and 11.10).
- The 18G needle entry point is just lateral or inferior to the transverse process, aiming at the L5 body. The needle is advanced to the desired depth, based on the patient's body habitus, using a tunnel vision technique. (In a thin individual, this is ~5cm).
- A 22G 150mm needle (bent 1 inch at the tip) is advanced via the 18G needle to touch the vertebral body, with the bent tip facing the vertebral body. This needle is then pulled back and rotated through 180° so that the curvature is facing outside. After advancement for 1 inch, it is again rotated through 180° to hug the vertebral body. Lateral and AP views are obtained to confirm the needle tip position just anterior to the L5 vertebral body.
- Low-volume tubing is attached to the 22G needle and contrast injected under continuous fluoroscopic view, followed by the therapeutic agent. This is to prevent accidental needle-tip movement while connecting and disconnecting the needle hub.
- The procedure is repeated on the opposite side.
- A total of 20–30mL LA, saline, and Depo-Medrone can be used. Neurolytic agents can be used, but a larger needle may be necessary depending on the agent (see 📖 Chapter 3, p. 30).

Transdiscal approach

- Prone position with a pillow under the pelvis to flatten the lumbar lordosis.
- Identify the L5/S1 interspace and square the vertebral endplates by a cephalic tilt.
- Rotate the C-arm obliquely to obtain a 'scottie dog' view. An 18G needle is then introduced parallel to the beam, aiming just in front of the superior articular process (the scottie dog's ear).
- Introduce a 22G needle is into the L5/S1 disc via the larger needle. If there is any doubt, radio-opaque contrast can be injected to confirm disc entry.
- Under a lateral view advance the needle slowly to exit the disc anteriorly. After AP and lateral confirmation of needle tip position, inject radio-opaque contrast under continuous fluoroscopy.
- This technique increases the risk of discitis. Addition of intradiscal antibiotics according to local guidelines can reduce this risk.

Advantages of the transdiscal approach

- Easier technically
- Minimal risk of organ puncture
- Low risk of intravascular injection
- Single-needle technique is possible.

Anterior approach

- Patient is positioned supine and 15° Trendelenburg.
- Identify body of the L5 vertebra using the AP view fluoroscopically.
- Insert a 22G 6mm needle in the midline perpendicular to the floor until it contacts the caudal two-thirds of the L5 vertebral body.
- After checking for blood on aspiration, confirm placement by injection of contrast and checking its spread in AP and lateral views under continuous fluoroscopy.
- Although not widely used, this technique is claimed to be technically easier and allows the use of a single injection.

Complications

- Bleeding from the common iliac vessels leading to a retroperitoneal haematoma.
- Intravascular injection.
- Neural complications (e.g. injury to cauda equina and exiting nerve roots). Placement of the needle too medially may result in epidural, subdural, or subarachnoid injection.
- Damage to pelvic visceral organs (e.g. bladder, ureter, kidney, and bowel) can occur.
- The transdiscal approach can result in discitis, disc rupture, or disc herniation.

Ganglion impar block

Anatomy
The ganglion impar (ganglion of Walther) is the terminal ganglion of the sympathetic chain that lies in front of the sacrococcygeal junction in the retroperitoneal space. It receives fibres from the lumbosacral sympathetic and parasympathetic nervous system.

Indications
- Perineal pain
- Sympathetic pain from rectum and genitalia
- Coccydynia, proctalgia fugax.

Contraindications
- Patient refusal
- Anticoagulation
- Local skin infection.

Procedure
The routes used for the ganglion impar block are shown in Fig. 11.14.

Sacrococcygeal route
- Prone position with a pillow under the pelvis.
- Lateral radiograph to view the sacrococcygeal junction (Fig. 11.15(a)).
- After local infiltration, a 22G needle is introduced via the sacrococcygeal junction and advanced just anterior to the junction.
- Contrast confirmation is followed by injection of LA with steroid (Fig. 11.15(b)).
- The same approach could be used with the patient in the lateral position.

Anococcygeal route
- Prone position with a pillow under the pelvis.
- Bent 22G needle to mimic the curvature of the coccyx.
- After local infiltration, the needle is introduced through the anococcygeal ligament to reach just anterior to sacroccocygeal joint.
- After contrast confirmation, LA and steroid can be injected.

Complications
- Bleeding
- Infection
- Rectal perforation
- Fistula formation.

Assessment
Assess for improvement in the pain scores both in the immediate post-operative period and in the follow-up clinic using pain diaries.

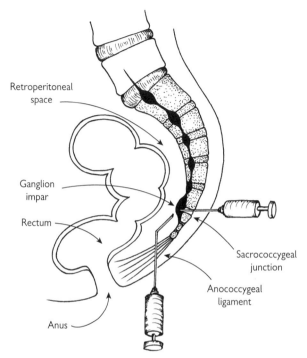

Fig. 11.14 The anococygeal and sacrococcygeal routes for performing the ganglion impar block.

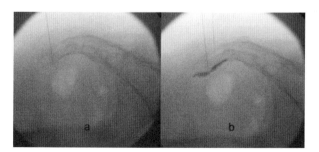

Fig. 11.15 (a) Lateral X-ray showing the needle through the sacro-coccygeal junction. (b) Good contrast spread anterior to the sacro-cocygeal junction. Another needle is in position for a caudal epidural.

Spinal interventions for cancer pain

M.L. Sharma

Intrathecal neurolysis for cancer pain

In this chapter we focus on intrathecal (IT) neurolytic blockade for terminal cancer pain. There are no controlled studies, and so the literature is observational, case reports and book chapters reflecting the opinions of experienced clinicians. Many other interventions including spinal RF procedures, continuous epidural analgesia, IT pumps, and open or percutaneous cordotomy have a role in carefully selected patients, but these are beyond the scope of this chapter.

IT neurolysis involves the destruction of nerve root axons or other spinal cord elements by a chemical (e.g. alcohol or phenol). Interruption of noci-ceptive pathways can produce excellent analgesia in a selected body area. IT neurolysis can be useful for terminally ill patients with pain in only a few dermatomes (e.g. for perineal or thoracic pain). This treatment is often accompanied by numbness or dysaesthetic symptoms which can be unpleasant. It has fallen out of favour because of improvements in pharmacological management of cancer pain and IT analgesia.

The technique requires careful patient selection, precision, and meticulous attention to detail. This is particularly true in the lumbar area where the space between the sensory and motor roots is virtually non-existent, which makes selective blocking of the sensory roots very difficult. In the thoracic area it is easier to produce segmental neurolysis of the posterior rami.

Indications

IT neurolysis can be used for perineal or pelvic pain caused by cancer that is refractory to conservative treatment including opioids, radiotherapy, and chemotherapy. It can be used for chest wall pain in one or two dermatomes (e.g. from secondaries). It is usually avoided in arm or leg pain for fear of causing motor weakness.

Contraindications

- Local or systemic infection
- Bleeding diathesis or uncorrectable anticoagulation
- Progressive neurological deficit
- Brain metastasis
- Established or impending spinal cord compression.

Agents used for intrathecal neurolysis

Phenol

The neurolytic effects of phenol are mediated by coagulation of proteins. The neurotoxic action is related to concentration. Phenol has a greater affinity for vascular tissue than for myelin phospholipids, and this may be of concern if it is injected close to vascular structures. Its high affinity for peri-neural blood vessels means that extreme care is needed with coeliac plexus block. It acts as an LA at low concentrations and as a neurolytic at higher concentrations. Because its local anaesthetic properties, no burning sensation is produced during injection; patients feel warmth, numbing, or dysaesthetic sensations. It is hyperbaric in mixtures of 4–10%; an aqueous mixture is a more potent neurolytic. Phenol 4% is comparable to alcohol 40%. It is available as a mixture with glycerol, in which it is highly soluble; it diffuses out slowly resulting in pronounced localized tissue effects. Use of a 20G spinal needle is helpful because of the viscosity of phenol in glycerol. It has a short-lived effect—neural degeneration takes 14 days and recovery about 14 weeks.

Alcohol

Alcohol exerts its neurolytic action by dehydration, with extraction of cholesterol, phospholipids, and cerebrosides. This leads to precipitation of mucoproteins and lipoproteins, resulting in sclerosis of nerve fibres and myelin sheaths. It is used in concentrations of 50–90%. Its specific gravity of 0.8 (CSF 1.1) means that it is hypobaric in relation to CSF. A tuberculin syringe is preferred and aliquots of 0.1mL are injected. The patient is told to expect severe localized burning pain for a few seconds after each injection and to report whether the burning pain occurs at, above, or below the level of pain.

Techniques

Hyperbaric phenol

Preparation

- Consent should include discussion of the likely success rate and potential complications. All patients must be warned about the risk of numbness, motor weakness, and dysaesthesiae. If phenol is being used for perineal pain, they should be warned about the possibility of sphincter control problems.
- If the patient has perineal pain, position them sitting. For chest wall pain, a lateral position is used with the painful side dependent. After injection of viscous phenol in glycerol, the patient is positioned so as to allow the neurolytic agent to flow preferentially towards the dorsal roots. This is achieved by using a 45° head-up tilt for perineal pain. If pain is in one side of perineum/pelvis, the patient is tilted to that side.
- Equipment includes a 20G spinal needle, a 1mL Luer lock syringe, and 5–10% viscous phenol in glycerol. Intravenous access is preferable.
- Strict asepsis is essential, including sterile skin preparation, surgical drapes, and surgical mask, gown, gloves, and hat.
- Some patients may be very frail or taking large amounts of medication, and they may need extra support to keep a steady position during the procedure.

Pelvic pain

The patient is positioned sitting on a trolley or operating table. Under aseptic conditions, a midline lumbar puncture is carried out with a 20G spinal needle at L3/4 or L4/5. Once a good flow of CSF is established, the patient is tilted backwards and 0.75–1.5mL of viscous phenol in glycerol is slowly injected over 2min. The volume injected depends on the strength of phenol in glycerol available (5–10%). The block may need repeating after 7 days if local disease is widespread. It is better to be judicious with the volume injected as the block can easily be repeated if necessary. The patient is positioned with a 45° head-up tilt on the trolley for 45min to allow the neurolytic to fix to nervous tissue. If pain is one-sided, the trolley is also tilted to that side by 15–20°. Patients usually report immediate pain relief as phenol has LA properties.

Chest wall pain

This is not as simple as a saddle block. Depending on the area involved, either a single-needle or multiple-needle technique can be used. The equipment and neurolytic are the same as as for a saddle block. It is advisable that the clinician undertaking the procedure understands that spinal nerves exit the vertebral column one or two levels below the point where they originate in spinal cord (Fig. 12.1). For example, to produce chemical neurolysis for the T5 dermatome, the spinal needle must be inserted at the T3/4 interspinous space. Knowledge of dermatomes (Fig. 12.2) is vital for the safe use of this technique. A lateral position with the painful side dependent is used (Fig. 12.3). The patient may be leaned backwards to allow the hyperbaric phenol to spread preferentially to the dorsal roots. A volume of 0.75–1.0mL of phenol in glycerol is needed for each dermatome involved. If the single-needle technique is being used, a larger volume of neurolytic may be required.

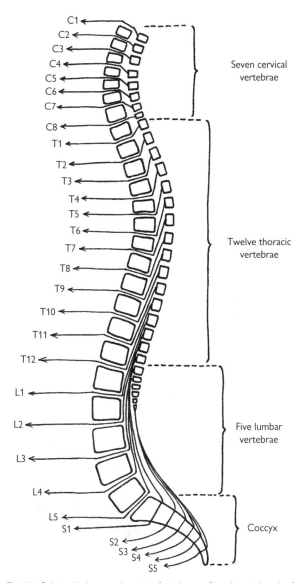

Fig. 12.1 Relationship between the origin of spinal nerves from the spinal cord and point of exit from spinal column.

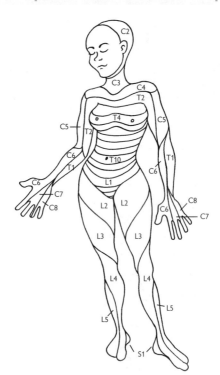

Fig. 12.2 Side view of dermatomes.

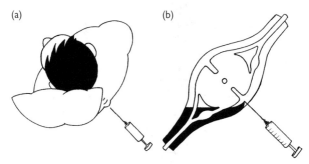

Fig. 12.3 Patient position for the use of phenol for thoracic chemical neurolysis.

Alcohol

Patient preparation, including consent, is the same as for IT phenol except for the patient's position during injection. Absolute alcohol is hypobaric in relation to CSF. The patient is positioned with painful side uppermost in relation to the point at which alcohol is to be injected into the CSF (Fig. 12.4). For thoracic neurolysis the patient may be leaned forward to allow alcohol to spread preferentially to the dorsal roots. For perineal pain the patient has to be positioned prone with pillows under the abdomen such that the sacrum is the highest point of spine. Usually 0.75–1.0mL of absolute alcohol is sufficient.

Tips

- A 20G spinal needle is preferable as it is difficult to push viscous phenol in glycerol through smaller needles.
- Luer lock syringe.
- If using absolute alcohol as the neurolytic agent, do not aspirate CSF into the syringe containing alcohol as it will crystallize the solution.

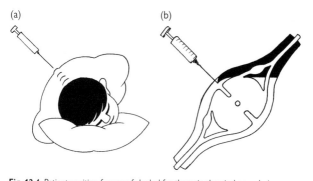

(a)   (b)

Fig. 12.4 Patient position for use of alcohol for thoracic chemical neurolysis.

Postoperative care

Aftercare

It is preferable to keep the patient in a palliative care/hospice environment for the first few days to allow down-titration of opioids and to assess the patient's response. It is unusual for patients to develop post-dural puncture headache. Occasionally the neurolytic block may have to be repeated after about a week if the initial response is partial.

Complications

- Numbness
- Motor weakness
- Dysaesthesia
- Sphincter control impairment
- Neuropathic pain
- Paraplegia
- Sexual dysfunction.

Further reading

British Pain Society (2010). *Cancer Pain Management*. Available online at: http://www. britishpainsociety.org/book_cancer_pain.pdf.

Candido K, Stevens RA (2003). Intrathecal neurolytic blocks for the relief of cancer pain. *Best Pract Res Clin Anaesthesiol* **17**: 407–28.

Lifshitz S, Debacker LJ, Buchsbaum HJ (1976). Subarachnoid phenol block for pain relief in gynaecologic malignancy. *Obstet Gynecol* **48**: 316–20.

Plancarte R, Alvarez J, Arrieta MA (2003). Interventional treatments of cancer pain. *Semin Pain Med* **1**: 34–42.

Slatkin NE, Reiner M (2003). Phenol saddle block at end of life: report of four cases and literature review. *Am J Hosp Palliat Care* **20**: 62–6.

Head and neck interventions

K.N. Shoukrey, R. Munglani, and M.L. Sharma

Sphenopalatine ganglion block

Introduction

Sluder's neuralgia was first described in 1908 and was treated with the sphenopalatine ganglion block (SPGB). Currently, SPGB is used for the relief of certain types of facial pain and headache. It has provided pain relief in patients when conventional pharmacological therapy has become less effective or has been completely ineffective.

Anatomy

The sphenopalatine ganglion (SPG), or pterygopalatine ganglion, is the largest group of neurons outside the cranial cavity. It is ~5mm in size and lies in the pterygopalatine fossa, which is ~1cm wide × 2cm high and resembles a vase on a lateral fluoroscopic view. The ganglion lies within the fossa and is located posterior to the middle nasal turbinate and a few millimetres deep to the lateral nasal mucosa. The fossa also contains the maxillary nerve and the maxillary artery with its multiple branches that pass more laterally in the fossa.

The pterygopalatine fossa has the following boundaries.

- Anterior: the posterior wall of the maxillary sinus
- Posterior: the medial plate of the pterygoid process
- Medial: the perpendicular plate of the palatine bone
- Superior: the sphenoid sinus
- Lateral: communicates with the infratemporal fossa
- Superolateral: the maxillary branch of the trigeminal nerve exits the cranial vault through the foramen rotundum

The SPG has a complex neural centre: it joins the maxillary branch of the trigeminal nerve via the pterygopalatine nerves, and it also joins the vidian nerve (nerve of the pterygoid canal) which is formed by the greater petrosal and deep petrosal nerves. The SPG is also in direct connection with the greater and lesser palatine nerves which give rise to superior, posterior, lateral nasal, and pharyngeal nerves. The SPG has sensory components from the maxillary nerve. They pass through the SPG and are distributed to the nasal membranes, the soft palate, and some parts of the pharynx. A few motor nerves may also be carried with the sensory trunks.

The autonomic components of the SPG are the most significant and are thought to play a significant role in a number of pain syndromes. The sympathetic component begins with upper thoracic pre-ganglionic sympathetic fibres forming the white rami communicantes, travelling in the sympathetic chain and synapsing with the post-ganglionic fibres in the superior cervical sympathetic ganglion. The post-ganglionic fibres then join the carotid nerves and travel via the deep petrosal nerve through the SPG on their way to the lacrimal gland and the nasal and palatine mucosa. The parasympathetic component has its pre-ganglionic origin in the superior salivatory nucleus and then travels through a portion of the facial nerve (cranial nerve (CN) VII) before forming the greater petrosal nerve which in turn joins the deep petrosal nerve that ends in the SPG.

Within the ganglion, the pre-ganglionic fibres synapse with their post-ganglionic cells and continue on to the nasal mucosa. One branch travels with the maxillary nerve to the lacrimal gland.

Indications

SPGB can be used for the following:

- acute migraine headache
- acute and chronic cluster headache
- facial neuralgias (sphenopalatine and trigeminal)
- status migrainosus
- atypical facial pain
- herpes zoster ophthalmicus.

RF procedures to the SPG:

- cancer pain
- headache and facial pain syndromes that fail to respond to conservative management including a repeated course of local blockade.

Contraindications

Absolute

- Patient refusal
- Allergy to LA
- Local infection
- Coagulopathy.

Relative

- Altered anatomy secondary to surgery, infection, or genetic variations
- Inability to obtain informed consent
- Inability by the patient to determine a cause-and-effect relationship for symptoms.

Technique

Lateral approach (trans-coronoid notch approach) under X-ray

SPGB via the lateral approach is accomplished by injection of LA onto the ganglion by placing of a needle through the coronoid notch (Figs. 13.1 and 13.2). It is also the best approach for RF to the SPG.

- The patient lies supine with the head inside the C-arm. Aseptic techniques, LA, and sedation are used as per local protocols.
- A lateral view of the upper cervical spine and the mandible is obtained and the head is rotated until the rami of the mandible are super-imposed on each other.
- The C-arm is moved slightly cephalad until the pterygopalatine fossa is visualized. It is located just posterior to the posterior aspect of the maxillary sinus and should resemble a vase when the two pterygo-palatine plates are superimposed on each another.
- A 22G 10cm needle is inserted under the zygoma and anterior to the ramus of the mandible.
- The needle is directed medial, cephalad, and towards the pterygo-palatine fossa (Fig. 13.1(a)).
- An AP view confirms that the needle is properly positioned (Fig. 13.1(b)).

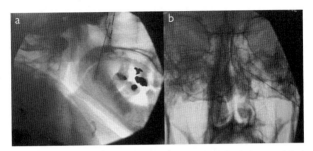

Fig. 13.1 (a) Lateral X-ray of an SPGB with the needle entering the pterygo-palatine fossa. The outline of the fossa has been enhanced. (b) AP view—the needle should come very close to the lateral nasal mucosa without penetrating it.

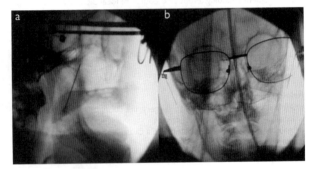

Fig. 13.2 In these (a) lateral and (b) AP X-rays the patient's spectacles have been left *in situ* and the mouth is open to give a clearer view of the anatomy.

The tip of the needle should be advanced until it is adjacent to the lateral nasal mucosa. If resistance is felt at any time, the needle must be slightly withdrawn and redirected. Avoid advancing the needle through the lateral nasal mucosa as this can lead to bleeding or infection.

After negative aspiration, 1–3mL of 0.5% L-bupivacaine and steroid is injected slowly. Further solution may be left along the needle insertion track.

RF lesioning

RF lesioning of the SPG can be either conventional or pulsed after a successful block has been produced with LA. It is accomplished by placing an RF needle in proximity to the SPG. Care must be taken to avoid inadvertent neurolysis of the maxillary nerve when performing conventional RF on the SPG because of the ability to localize the SPG more accurately by stimulation. The lateral approach is probably the safest option if destruction of the SPG is desired.

- An insulated 22G 10cm RF needle with a 5–10mm active tip is used.
- A sensory stimulation at 0.5–0.7 V should induce parasthesia at the root of the nose. If stimulation is felt in the upper teeth or the side of the face, one may be too close to the maxillary nerve and the needle should be redirected more caudad and medially (i.e. inwards towards the nose). If stimulation is felt in the area of the hard palate, one may be too close to the greater and lesser palatine nerves and the tip should be directed more posterior.
- RF lesioning is performed for 70–90s at 80°C. Two or three lesions are usually made after 2–3mL of LA is first injected.
- Pulsed RF (3–6min) at <42°C may also be performed with or without injecting any LA first.

Complications

Blockade of the SPG is not a benign procedure. Table 13.1 shows the possible side effects and complications and the reasons for their occurrence.

Table 13.1 Side effects and complications of SPGB

Side effect/complication	Reason for occurrence
Epistaxis and infection	Needle advanced too far so that it is pushed through the lateral nasal wall via the lateral approach
Haematoma formation	Puncture of the large venous plexus overlying the pterygopalatine fossa or the maxillary artery
LA toxicity	Significant systemic absorption of LA due to high vascularity
Longer-term hypo-aesthesia of the soft palate may occur even with well-placed lesions and is usually of no consequence. Transient (usually) hyper-aesthesia of the palate, maxilla, or the posterior pharynx may occur with RF lesioning	Direct injury or lesioning of the maxillary and mandibular nerves
Orthostatic hypotension	Sympathetic blockade
Reflex bradycardia (during RF lesioning)	May be caused by a reflex resembling the oculocardiac reflex
Impairment of ipsilateral lacrimation or nasal/palatal mucus production	Destruction of the secretomotor function of the SPG or mechanical injury to structures superficial to the pterygopalatine fossa (parotid gland and branches of the facial nerve)
Allergic reaction	Allergy to LA or steroid

Percutaneous interventions for trigeminal neuralgia

Introduction

Percutaneous trigeminal ganglion level interventions are very effective for medically refractory trigeminal neuralgia. RF and balloon micro-compression of the Gasserian ganglion are neuroablative procedures. Following these procedures, patients usually experience numbness in the trigeminal nerve distribution for a variable period of time. These procedures should be offered for trigeminal neuralgia rather than for atypical facial pain. If an MRI scan shows neurovascular compression at the trigeminal root entry zone on the affected side, microvascular decompression should be considered as it has an excellent long-term outcome.

Anatomical considerations

The trigeminal nerve is a mixed nerve consisting primarily of sensory neurons. It exits the brain on the lateral surface of the pons, and enters the trigeminal ganglion within a few millimetres. The trigeminal ganglion corresponds to the dorsal root ganglion of a spinal nerve. Three major branches emerge from the trigeminal ganglion. Each branch innervates a different dermatome and exits the cranium through a different foramen. The first division (CN V1, ophthalmic nerve) exits the cranium through the superior orbital fissure, entering the orbit to innervate the globe and skin in the area above the eye and forehead. The second division (CN V2, maxillary nerve) exits through the foramen rotundum into a space posterior to the orbit, the pterygopalatine fossa. It supplies the middle third of the face. The third division (CN V3, mandibular nerve) exits the cranium through an oval hole, the foramen ovale. It supplies the lower third of the face. If the needle trajectory is too posterior, it may enter the foramen lacerum through which the carotid artery passes. If the needle trajectory is too anterior, it may enter the orbital cavity, leading to retrobulbar haemorrhage. If the needle is too medial and deep, injury to the cavernous sinus and the cranial nerve supply to the eyeball may occur.

Indications for RF/balloon microcompression

- Medically refractory trigeminal neuralgia and MRI scan not showing neurovascular compression.
- It may be offered to patients with a positive MRI scan if the patient is unwilling or unfit to have surgery (microvascular decompression). It is very useful for multiple sclerosis patients suffering from trigeminal neuralgia.

RF thermocoagulation of the Gasserian ganglion

- Needs patient cooperation with sensory stimulation and re-testing after the RF lesion
- It is not recommended for V1 (ophthalmic) neuralgia

Balloon microcompression

- Preferred for V1 (ophthalmic) neuralgia
- Patient (operator) preference to have the procedure under general anaesthesia.

Contraindications

- Local or systemic infection
- Bleeding diathesis or anticoagulation
- Numbness in painful area (trigeminal neuropathy)

RF thermocoagulation of the Gasserian ganglion

Preparation

- Consent includes discussion of the likely success rate and potential complications. All patients must be warned about the risk of numbness and potential jaw weakness. All patients should have brain MRI to rule out neurovascular compression at the trigeminal root entry zone, tumour, multiple sclerosis, or any other central causes.
- Prepare the patient as for general anaesthesia.
- Position the patient supine on a radiolucent table with a thin pillow under the head. Clear X-ray images are needed as identification of the foramen ovale is essential.
- Equipment needed: RF lesion generator; 22G 100mm RF needle with a 5mm active tip; thermocouple probe for sensory stimulation and RF lesioning; LA; simple equipment for sensory examination after the heat lesion.
- Strict asepsis is essential. It is usual to administer one dose of prophylactic antibiotic according to local guidance.
- An anaesthetist must be present to monitor the patient and administer general anaesthesia.

Technique

- The C-arm should be positioned with ~45° caudal tilt and 15–30° ipsilateral oblique tilt to identify the foramen ovale. Minor adjustments may be needed to define its margins clearly.
- Usually the foramen is visualized just medial to the condyle of the mandible (Fig. 13.3).
- It may be beneficial for beginners to have experienced colleagues or an experienced radiologist/radiographer in theatre.

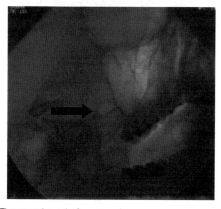

Fig. 13.3 The arrow shows the foramen ovale.

- The needle entry point lies just laterally to the angle of the mouth (2–3cm). The skin and subcutaneous tissues over this point are infiltrated with LA.
- An RF needle is advanced carefully towards the foramen ovale (Fig. 13.4). If targeting the second or third division, enter ~2cm away from the angle of the mouth, aiming for the middle third of foramen ovale. If targeting the first division, start ~3cm away from the angle of the mouth, aiming for the medial third of the foramen ovale. It is usually possible to have tactile sensation while passing through foramen ovale. This can be very painful and general anaesthesia may be needed at this stage.
- Perform motor stimulation at 2Hz. If there is masseter movement at low sensory thresholds (<0.5V), advance the needle by 2mm and retest until these movements disappear. Check the needle position with a lateral X-ray view. Stop the anaesthetic, wake the patient, and perform sensory stimulation at 50Hz. Try to produce paraesthesiae in the affected division of the trigeminal nerve at low thresholds (0.05–0.2V). CSF may drip through the needle; this is entirely acceptable.
- If paraesthesiae occur in the correct division of the trigeminal nerve, create an RF lesion at 65°C for 60s. The patient will need to be anaesthetized for this lesion as it is very painful. After the lesion, check sensory testing in the affected area of the face to see whether the patient has developed numbness. If not, the RF lesion will need to be repeated at 70°C and even up to 75°C until there is objective evidence of numbness.

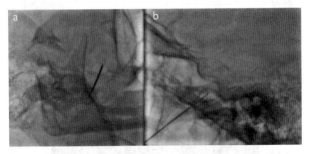

Fig. 13.4 (a) 22G RF cannula advanced through the foramen ovale. (b) Lateral view showing the final position of the RF needle.

Pearls of wisdom
- After the RF needle has been inserted through the foramen ovale, check the depth of needle insertion with a lateral view. The needle should not be inserted beyond the clival line as this can be very dangerous.
- Try to avoid inserting the RF needle through the buccal mucosa as this can introduce infection. Prevent this by inserting one finger into the mouth when initially inserting the RF needle.
- Clear biplanar imaging facilities help with visualization of the foramen ovale.
- A very cooperative patient is needed for this procedure.

- This procedure needs close cooperation between the operator and anaesthetist as the patient may need multiple sleep–wake cycles to produce numbness in the affected division of trigeminal nerve.

Trigeminal balloon microcompression

- This may be preferable in patients who cannot tolerate RF lesioning of the Gasserian ganglion. Consent, preparation, position, and image guidance to visualize the foramen ovale are as for the RF technique
- Equipment: 14G cannula; 4FG Fogarty embolectomy catheter; radio-opaque contrast
- The procedure is carried out under general anaesthesia as the patient's cooperation is not needed
- A 14G needle is passed under X-ray guidance up to the level of the foramen ovale (Fig. 13.5(a)). The needle does not need to go as deep as in the RF technique (Fig. 13.6(a))
- A 4FG Fogarty embolectomy catheter is introduced through the 14G needle. The balloon is inflated with 0.6–0.8 mL of Omnipaque 300 for 1min and then deflated for 1min. Two more inflation–deflation cycles are repeated
- A pear-shaped inflated balloon reflects effective compression of the Gasserian ganglion (Fig. 13.6(a)). It is reassuring to see a medial projection of the inflated balloon on an AP view (Fig. 13.6(b))
- At the end of procedure the needle and Fogarty balloon are withdrawn together. Trying to remove the balloon through the needle may result in shearing of bits of balloon and these may be left behind.

Pearls of wisdom

- The Fogarty balloon should be de-aired to facilitate effective compression of the trigeminal ganglion
- The 14G needle should be introduced only up to the level of the foramen ovale and no further
- Transient bradycardia or even asystole may be observed with balloon inflation or when the needle is inserted through the foramen.

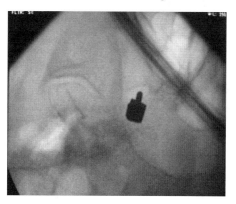

Fig. 13.5 Balloon compression: 14G needle advanced through foramen ovale.

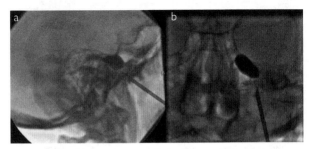

Fig. 13.6 Balloon compression: (a) pear shape of inflated balloon in Meckel's cave; (b) AP view showing medial trajectory of the inflated balloon.

Aftercare following RF or balloon compression
The patient needs the usual postoperative care and can usually be discharged the next day. With careful planning, the procedure can be performed as a day-case. The patient may need simple analgesics for postoperative pain. It is good practice to do a neurological examination the day after and document numbness, jaw weakness, and the presence or absence of a corneal reflex.

Complications of RF or Gasserian ganglion/balloon micro-compression
- Temporary jaw weakness (more common with balloon micro-compression)
- Cheek haematoma (settles quickly)
- Unpleasant dysaesthesia
- Anaesthesia dolorosa (1–4%, more common with RF)
- Cranial nerve palsy (temporary).

Very rare complications
- Corneal ulceration
- Retrobulbar hemorrhage
- Carotid artery puncture
- Intracranial haemorrhage
- Meningitis.

Further reading
Erdine S, Ozyalcin NS, Cimen A, Celik M, Talu GK, Disci R (2007). Comparison of pulsed RF with conventional RF in the treatment of idiopathic trigeminal neuralgia. *Eur J Pain* **11**: 309–13.

Mullan S, Lichtor T (1983). Percutaneous micro compression of the trigeminal ganglion for trigeminal neuralgia. *J Neurosurg* **59**: 1007–12.

Nurmikko TJ, Eldridge PR (2001). Trigeminal neuralgia: pathophysiology, diagnosis and current treatment. *Br J Anaesth* **87**: 117–32.

Skirving DJ, Dan NG (2001). A 20-year review of percutaneous balloon compression of the trigeminal ganglion. *J Neurosurg* **94**: 913–17.

Tatli M, Satici O, Kanpolat Y, Sindou M (2008). Various surgical modalities for trigeminal neuralgia: literature study of respective long-term outcomes. *Acta Neurochirurg* **150**: 243–55.

Medicolegal issues and interventional pain management

K. Simpson

Medicolegal issues

Doctors in pain medicine may be involved in medicolegal matters for many reasons. They may be a witness to fact or an expert witness in civil or criminal matters. Unfortunately, they may also be involved after an adverse event with their own patient that results in litigation against the individual or their organization. This chapter deals with expert witness work and relies on the author's experience of medicolegal work in the UK over the past 15 years as an expert witness in civil matters (personal injury and medical negligence), criminal matters, and fitness to practice cases heard by the General Medical Council (GMC). The chapter will focus on general issues with regard to being an expert witness and it will give some personal views. It must be remembered that specific points of law vary depending upon the place of practice; for example, Scottish, Welsh, Irish, European, American, and Australasian systems differ. However, the principles of being a good expert witness are universal.

Pain medicine specialists who are involved in medicolegal work should have a basic understanding of the rules of litigation that apply to the area in which they practice. In the UK there are Civil Procedure Rules and Criminal Procedure Rules. All expert witnesses must be familiar with these rules and must understand their duties as an expert witness. These duties are clearly set out by the GMC; failure to follow GMC guidance in this area can lead to fitness to practice concerns in just the same way as can deficiencies in clinical care. Since 2011 experts in the UK have lost their previous immunity; this has implications for practice and indemnity. Experts owe a duty to exercise reasonable skill and care to those instructing them and to comply with GMC professional codes of practice in all areas. Experts must provide opinions that are independent regardless of the pressures of litigation. If there is a conflict of interest, this must be stated before taking instructions. If this only becomes apparent later it must be disclosed. In the author's view, experts should try to avoid taking cases that involve their own patients or health-care professionals whom they know well. They must confine their opinion to matters that are material to the issues and provide an opinion only in relation to those areas that are within their expertise. Confidential information must not be disclosed other than to the parties involved in the proceedings. Exceptions are if a subject consents (if there are no other restrictions on disclosure), if the expert is obliged to disclose by law, a court, or a tribunal, or if their overriding duty to the court and the administration of justice demands disclosure. Experts must be familiar with information governance issues (e.g freedom of information and data protection legislation).

The British Medical Association (BMA) and various expert witness organizations provide useful information and fact sheets about many important medicolegal issues. Many organizations provide training for experts and this is highly recommended. This should include education about general principles of law relating to medical care, report writing, conferences with other experts or counsel, and appearing as an expert witness in court. It is as important to have adequate medical defence insurance for medicolegal work as it is for clinical work. Pain medicine specialists taking on medicolegal work must ensure that they have adequate training, time, and administrative support to manage their affairs.

Civil Procedure Rules

The 50th update of the Civil Procedure Rules (CPR), October 2009, is available online at www.justice.gov.uk.

The rules in civil litigation have several parts. It is good practice for all doctors to be familiar with these, whether or not they are involved in medicolegal work. The most relevant are CPR Part 1 which concerns the overriding objectives and CPR Part 2 which concerns practice direction.

CPR Part 1: overriding objectives

These rules have objectives that enable the court to deal with all cases justly. The rules ensure that, as far as practicable, all parties are on equal footing. The rules are there to save expense and deal with each case in a manner that is proportionate to costs, importance, complexity, and the financial position of each party. These rules should ensure that all cases are dealt with expeditiously and fairly. It is important that experts understand that their duty is to the court and that they must help the court to further the overriding objectives of CPR Part 1. The expert's primary duty is not to the party who has engaged or paid them. Their duty does not involve supporting the complainant or defendant; an expert must avoid straying into the role of advocate for either party. The court has a duty to manage cases; there are practices and procedures for active case management. These are designed to encourage the parties to cooperate with each other in the conduct of proceedings, identify issues early, and decide promptly about those issues that need investigation and on the order of business. The rules are designed to help parties settle the case. The court is responsible for fixing timetables and controlling the progress of the case. It is important that experts appreciate their overriding duty to the court and that, once they take on a case, there is a requirement to comply with all court directions. Medicolegal work can be time consuming and requires flexibility; although court appearances are few, their timetabling is now very strict. Experts are obliged to attend court if called upon to do so.

CPR Part 35: experts and assessors

These rules are designed to restrict expert evidence to that which is reasonably required to resolve proceedings. The overriding principle of fairness and justice in CPR Part 1 remains paramount. However, Part 35 tends to limit the use of expert evidence to reduce costs and save expert time; this is largely a good thing. Experts may be appointed to assist the court on behalf of the claimant/complainant or the defendant, or as a single joint expert (instructed on behalf of two or more parties including the claimant or complainant). The expert must help the court on matters only within their expertise; this duty overrides any obligation to the person from whom the expert has received instructions or by whom they will be paid. All expert evidence should be independent and not influenced by the pressures of litigation. The expert has a duty to assist the court by providing objective opinions on matters only within their expertise. They should consider all the facts and make it clear that these are separate from their opinion. An expert must alert the instructing parties when an issue or question falls outside their expertise or if they have not had sufficient information to form an opinion. The court has the power to restrict expert evidence. No party can call an expert without the court's permission; this is granted after the instructing party has identified what expert evidence is required and, where practicable, from whom. An expert has the right to ask the court for directions, but in the author's experience it is usually the case that direct communication with the instructing parties is the best way forward.

Most expert evidence is given as a written report that must comply with the directions of CPR Part 35. The report must deal with all the instructions, whether written or oral; it must clearly separate facts from opinion. The report should be addressed to the court and give details of the expert's qualifications and experience; providing a mini-CV as an appendix is useful. The report should set out any examinations, measurements, and tests, and should state who did them. When there is a range of opinion, this should be summarized and the reasons given for the expert's own opinion. In civil matters the standard of proof is either by a preponderance of evidence or by clear and convincing evidence. These are lower burdens of proof than in criminal matters for obvious reasons. A preponderance of evidence means that one side has more evidence in its favour than the other, even by the smallest degree, i.e. the evidence shows that the event is 'more likely than not'. The crucial issue is whether an event or outcome is more likely, i.e. 51% likely. This may be difficult for medical experts and feels somewhat artificial. As scientists, doctors often consider results of clinical trials where the probability is $p <0.05$, i.e. a 95% likelihood; this is not what a court is considering in civil matters. Sometimes the expert just has to 'grasp the nettle' and make a decision based on experience.

A summary of conclusions should be included in all reports; this is sometimes best placed at the beginning of a report to allow the court to gain a sense of the direction of the expert's thinking. If, when forming an opinion, the expert relies on publications, these should be appended in full rather than abstract form. Standard textbooks are often preferred rather than obscure references. A report or written evidence must be accurate, so reasonable steps must be taken to verify information. At the end of the report there must be a statement that the expert understands and has complied with their duty to the court; the form of words is as prescribed by CPR Part 35. If the expert is acting as a single joint expert, the report must be disclosed simultaneously to all parties.

Part 35.6 allows a party to put written questions to an expert about their report within 28 days after the report has been served. The questions must be only for verification of the report, unless the court gives permission or the other parties agree to supplementary questions. When a party submits questions to an expert they must, at the same time, send a copy to all relevant parties, and any response must also be disclosed to all parties. The court may direct that a discussion between experts occurs in a set timescale to produce a joint statement. This is to allow experts (usually but not always of like disciplines) to identify and discuss issues and where possible reach an agreement. The court may specify what issues the experts need to discuss and there may be an agreed agenda. The contents of the discussion are privileged. The purpose of the discussion is to reach a consensus about points agreed and points disputed; the joint statement is not requested to pressurize one of the parties to change their opinion. These expert meetings are not usually attended by legal representatives. If, after producing a report, an expert's view changes for any reason, they must communicate this to all parties immediately and, when appropriate, to the court.

Rules in criminal litigation

The 8th update of the Criminal Procedure Rules (CrimPR), October 2009, is available online at www.justice.gov.uk.

It is unusual for pain medicine specialists to be involved in criminal proceedings. However, expert witness evidence is occasionally needed in these circumstances. CrimPR Part 1 has the overriding objective that criminal cases are dealt with justly, including acquitting the innocent and convicting the guilty. CrimPR Part 1 covers dealing with prosecution and defence early, recognizing the rights of the defendant, and respecting the interests of witnesses, victims, and jurors. It states that cases must be dealt with efficiently and expeditiously, appropriate information should be available in court, and cases should be dealt with taking into account the gravity of the offence, the complexity of issues, consequences for the defendant, and the needs of other cases. Each participant, including the expert witnesses, must prepare and conduct the case in accordance with these overriding objectives. The duties of an expert to the court and the structure and contents of an expert's report are similar to those in a civil case. In criminal cases the test of evidence is 'beyond reasonable doubt'. This is the highest standard of proof that must be met by the prosecution's evidence in a criminal matter. It means that no other logical explanation can be derived from the facts except that the defendant committed the crime. This level of evidence must establish a particular point to a moral certainty and show that it is beyond dispute that any reasonable alternative is possible. The statement of truth in criminal cases is also a little different. The form of words in the statement of truth in civil and criminal cases is prescribed and cannot be altered.

It is essential that experts keep accurate records of information relied upon and on which they based their opinions. It is particularly important in criminal cases that experts keep a log of evidence reviewed. They should have a method for cataloguing and retaining this data for the appropriate period. In all legal work, confidential handling of evidence is vital and is a professional responsibility. All data protection principles apply. Experts must take all reasonable steps to make sure that appropriate consent for disclosure of information has been obtained (e.g. from the patient or claimant to whom the data refer); if this is not clear, the data must be sent back to the instructing team for clarification. Experts must take all reasonable steps to ensure that relevant materials are kept secure whilst in their possession. At the conclusion of cases it is the practice of some experts to return all evidence to the instructing party. Alternatively, the material can disposed of confidentially at the end of the case or at a time specified by the instructing party.

GMC guidelines on acting as an expert witness

The GMC core guidance document for doctors Good Medical Practice (www.GMC-UK.org) sets out the principles that underpin good medical care. When a doctor acts as an expert witness, they take on a different role. However, the principles of good medical practice as set out by the GMC apply just as much as when doctors act in their clinical role. The GMC guidance sets out the position of doctors with regard to personal integrity. The document clearly states how these principles apply in expert witness practice and lists sources of information and advice. It must be recognized that persistent failure or serious misconduct in this area puts registration at risk just as much as when these problems occur in clinical practice.

Pearls of wisdom for work as an expert witness

- Understand that your role is to assist the court only in areas within your expertise.
- Keep up to date in your area.
- Ensure that you understand exactly what issues you are being asked to address and what is required of you.
- Communicate regularly with your instructing solicitors.
- If a case has no hope of succeeding, tell the solicitors sooner rather than later!
- Less is more—judges want succinct reports.
- When providing written reports or giving evidence, restrict your statements to where you have relevant knowledge or direct experience. If a question falls outside your area, make this clear immediately.
- You are often providing advice for people who do not come from a medical background so your terminology should be clear.
- Provide a balanced opinion. State the facts on which you have based your opinion and provide relevant literature if necessary.
- If you give an opinion without the opportunity to examine an individual, explain why you have accepted an instruction with these limitations. Try to avoid this unless the person has died.
- If you change your opinion, you must tell the instructing parties and, if necessary, the court.
- Obtain some training on how to write reports and how to conduct yourself in conference and in court.
- Be honest, objective, and impartial, and you will not go wrong!

Further reading

Academy of Experts. *Experts' Declaration, Code of Practice for Expert Witnesses: Protocol for the Instruction of Experts to Give Evidence in Civil Claims.* http://www.academy-experts.org.
British Medical Association. *Expert Witness Guidance.* www.bma.org.uk/ap.nsf/Content/ Expertwitness.
Civil Evidence Act (1995). www.opsi.gov.uk/ACTS/acts1995/Ukpga_19950038_en_1.htm.
Civil Procedure Rules and the Criminal Procedure Rules. http://www.justice.gov.uk/procedure.htm.
Criminal Justice Act (2003). www.opsi.gov.uk/acts/acts2003/20030044.htm.
Expert Witness Institute. *Experts' Declaration, Code of Practice, Experts' Protocol, Model Form of Reports in Civil and Criminal Proceedings.* http://www.ewi.org.uk.
Society of Expert Witnesses. http://www.sew.org.uk.

Index